INTERMITTENT FASTING FOR WOMEN OVER 50

The Ultimate Simple Guide to Boost Metabolism and Weight Loss, Detox Your Body, and Increase Your Energy, Including a Tasty and Easy-to-Make Recipe Section

Scarlett Krieger

© Copyright 2021 - All rights reserved

Table Of Contents

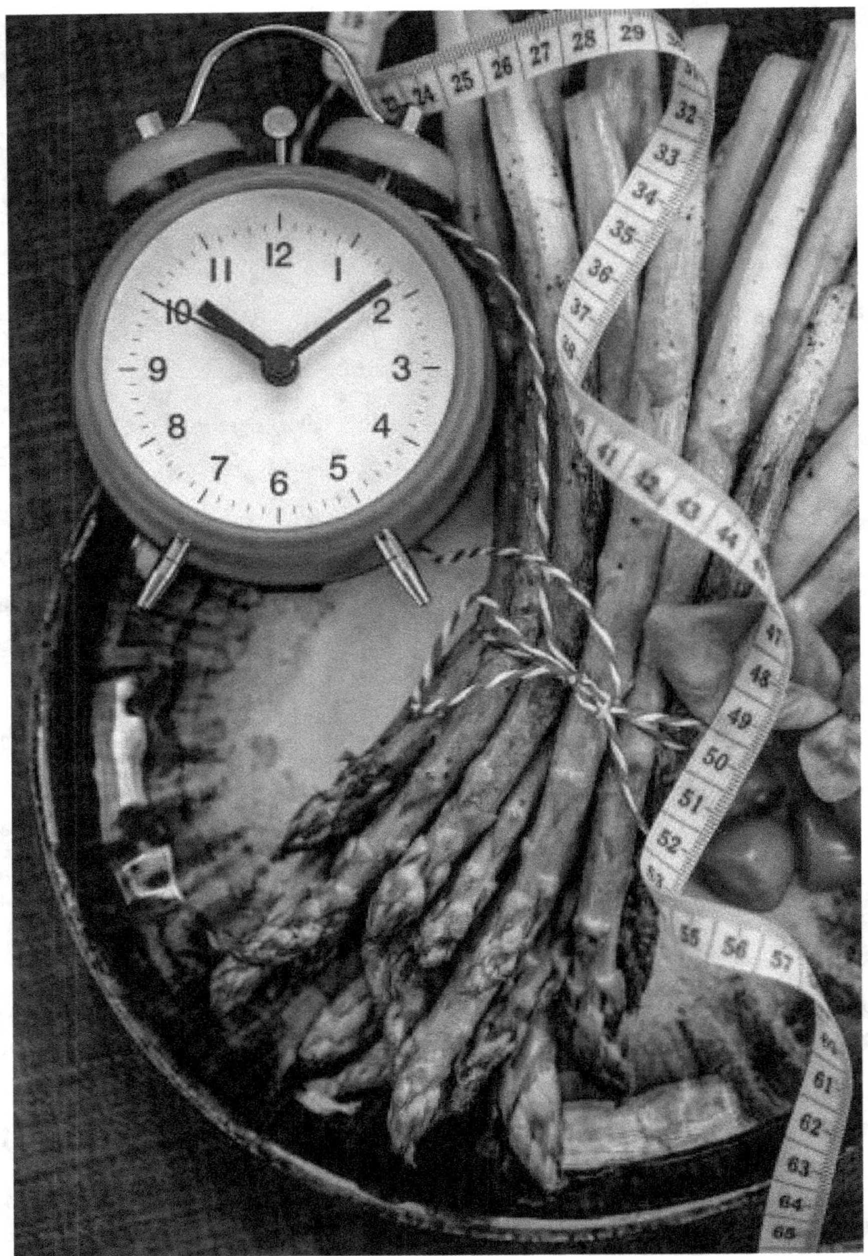

Introduction

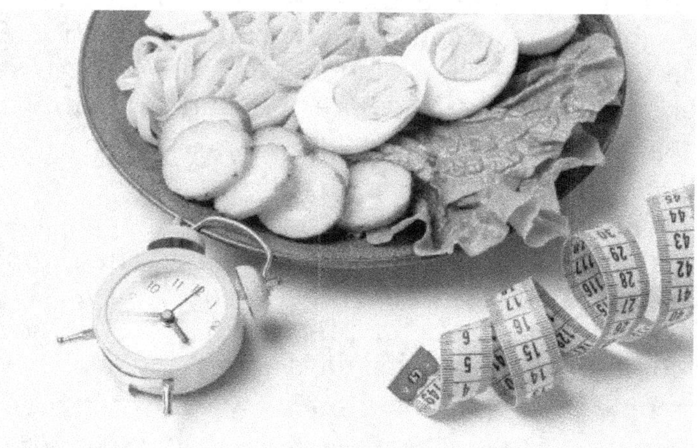

Women over 50 have unique needs and lifestyles that are different from women of other age groups. When we hear about fasting, it's usually for weight loss or for people who are in their teens or early 20s. But intermittent fasting may have a place in the lives of mature women as well.

The word "fasting" typically gets a bad rap. One morning, you might have dared to skip breakfast; the next, you find yourself scrounging for something at lunch that will push you past the 2-hour mark. That's fasting?

Intermittent fasting can benefit you by improving your body composition, downregulating inflammation and reducing calorie intake while still giving you plenty of energy to do all the things you enjoy doing every day. There's no need to fear starvation mode or going hungry! You will be eating just as many calories as you normally would, but with less food volume and more nutrient density.

Enter intermittent fasting (IF), a radical concept that is growing in popularity and changing preconceptions about what it means to go hungry. The term "intermittent" refers to periods of time when no food is consumed, which can range from 12 hours up to 72 hours. IF is also sometimes known as time-restricted feeding or eat-stop-eat.

Proponents of IF believe the practice benefits weight loss, longevity, blood sugar control and cognitive function. There's evidence to back up their claims. Here are eight reasons to think about trying it—if you're a healthy adult who isn't pregnant or breastfeeding, of course.

1. You'll lose weight.

Intermittent fasting is one of several strategies known to boost metabolism and promote fat loss. When your body doesn't get food for an extended period every day, it ramps up its fat-burning processes in preparation for the next meal (which could be hours or even days away).

Many people shed pounds simply by knowing they're less likely to overeat later. The key is not to overcompensate with extra food during the feeding window.

2. You could live longer.

In October 2014, a study published in the Journal of the American Medical Association reported that people who practiced IF were less likely to die from any cause over a 30-year period compared with those who didn't follow this eating pattern. Those who ate nothing every day had the highest risk of mortality, while those who followed a pattern that included one to two days of fasting per week were the healthiest.

3. You could improve your blood sugar control.

Limiting how often you eat can help keep blood sugar on an even keel, which is especially important for people with diabetes. One study found that women who practiced daily IF and ate only dinner were about half as likely to develop type 2 diabetes over a 4-year period compared with those who ate all day long. Eating only breakfast and lunch didn't have the same protective effect, however.

4. You could reduce disease risk.

In addition to the possibility of living longer, IF delivers other anti-aging benefits. For instance, some studies suggest that it can help control inflammation and oxidative stress—two factors in many chronic diseases. One study showed that when humans fasted for two days every month, their levels of oxidative stress decreased. IF may also prompt stem cells to differentiate into new blood cells—a process that could keep you healthier and more active as you get older.

5. You can improve your brain function—and possibly prevent Alzheimer's disease and other neurological disorders.

Fasting may also protect against oxidative stress and inflammation, which are linked with conditions like Alzheimer's disease. Fasting for 12 to 24 hours can also stimulate growth hormone production —a hormone vital to preserving brain function and warding off cognitive decline as you get older. The same goes for increasing ketone levels, which your body produces when it burns fat for fuel. Ketones act as an antioxidant in the brain, where they may help protect against neurodegenerative disorders like Parkinson's disease or Alzheimer's disease.

The bottom line? If you're looking for a way to reduce your calorie intake over time, IF could be a good option for you. Just keep in mind that there's no one right way to fast—you have many different options with varying benefits and drawbacks.

CHAPTER 1:

What is Fasting?

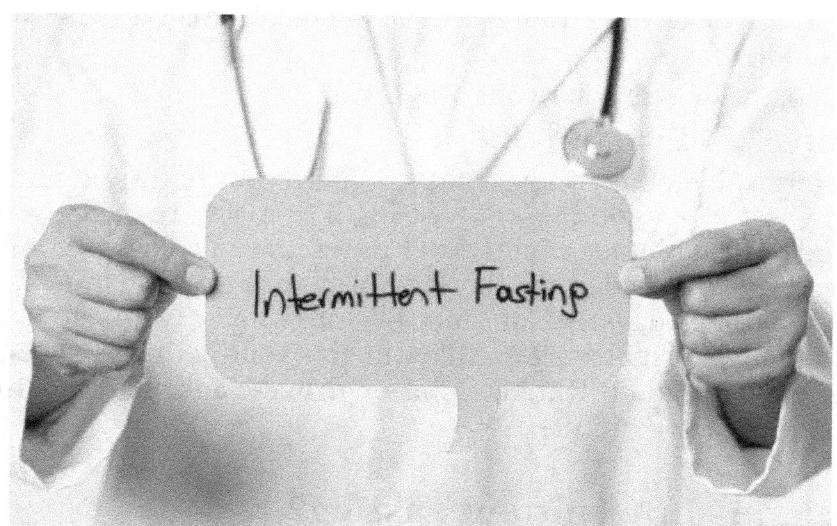

What Is Fasting?

Fasting is the act of limiting one's admission of nourishment for a while, normally under 24 hours. The reasons why individuals decide to fast are generally fluctuated. In this book, we will discuss fasting with an end goal to improve one's well-being, diminish the danger of illness and accomplish or keep a solid body weight.

Fasting can be used at any time during the year. Most of us are familiar with the idea of fasting during the Holy month of Ramadan (it requires total abstinence from food and water), but there are other types of fasting, such as intermittent fasting, which can help you get fit in different ways — it's not just about getting rid of fat!

There's something incredibly personal about every fast. So how do you get started?

Ask yourself: why do you want to fast?

To lose weight? To be healthier and feel amazing? To concentrate better at work or school? Or maybe to love and appreciate food more by taking a step back from it for a while.

It's important to have your goal in mind when starting out— the clarity will make all the difference. And if you're fasting for a specific health reason, make sure you talk to your doctor first to make sure there are no medical reasons why you shouldn't fast.

(Also, make sure you're not pregnant!)

Have Your Mind Set

Before you embark on your fast, prepare your body and mind. The best way to do this is by easing into it. Try reducing your food or drink intake slightly over the course of a few days. And once you've decided on the length of time you'd like to fast (e.g., 2 to 7 days), then start by introducing yourself to it gradually, in small stages. This will give your body a chance to get used to going without food or drink— and give you the confidence to continue.

What Is Intermittent Fasting?

Intermittent Fasting (IF) is an eating practice and diet routine that includes fasting for timeframes, at that point eating for timeframes, and pushing through this consistently. As the name states, you are fasting intermittently by burning through times of eating and not eating (fasting). These times of fasting and eating can differ. Intermittent Fasting doesn't have any limitations about what you can and can't eat, yet essentially when you can eat them.

The timeframes are normally somewhere near twelve hours of each, cycled each day. This strategy is like what you would likely ordinarily do, where you fast short-term while you are dozing, yet the long stretches of fasting are only somewhat more than expected. Different instances of intermittent fasting systems could be fasting for 16 hours in a day and then an eating window of 8 hours. When all is said in done, when you practice IF, you will isolate your day or your week into eating and fasting areas of time, which will rehash either consistently or consistently. With this kind of fasting, you can ingest fluids that have zero calories like water, espresso tea, and any others with no caloric substance. Simply be certain that adding sugar to your espresso or dark tea will invalid your fast.

Regarding well-being and strategies, including the body, no strategy will work for everybody in precisely the same manner. With regards to the body, everybody will respond contrastingly and will show various changes on its very own course of events. At the point when you are taking a stab at something new with an end goal to evoke changes from your body, you should remember that your body is special and personal. There are various approaches to fast and various thoughts of what are the best ways. Attempting things with an adaptable mentality will help you to find the way that turns out best for you.

CHAPTER 2:

A Brief History of Fasting

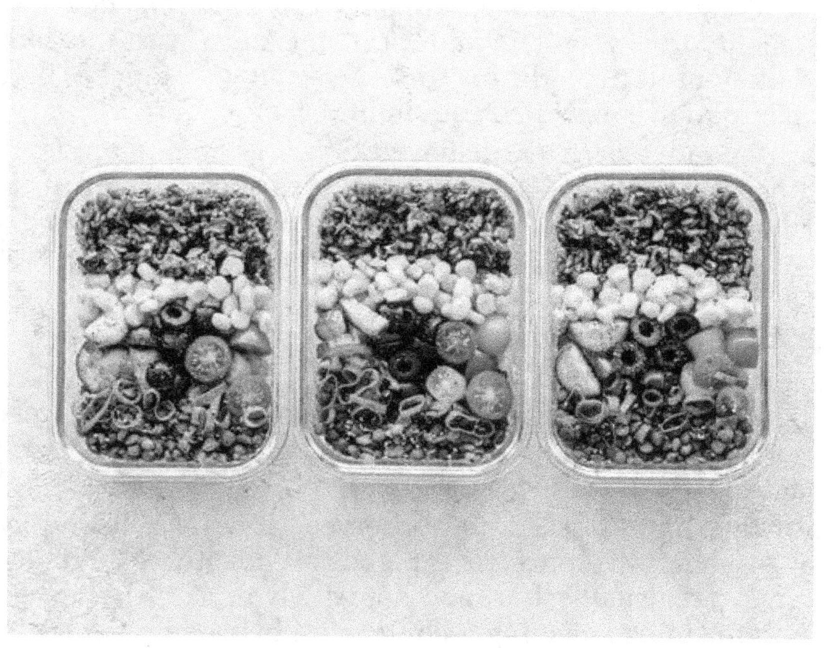

In many cultures, fasting is a practice that dates back thousands of years. Throughout history, fasting has had various meanings depending on the religion and culture in which it was practiced. Cultures have employed some form of fasting for religious reasons to achieve self-mastery or spiritual enlightenment—even as a form of political protest.

Fasting is not something new. Humans have been practicing various forms of fasting since ancient times, dating back to the time when we first moved away from living purely by hunting and gathering into communities with agriculture.

Our hunter-gatherer ancestors lived almost exclusively on meat and had to hunt for food every day. If a situation arose in which it became more advantageous to stay put in one place, humans would have been able to survive on the food they stored, but only for a short period of time.

When humans first started settling in communities with agriculture, their lifestyle shifted towards consuming foods that were far less perishable. This meant that those who could hold out longer would have been more likely to survive and pass along their genes. Over time these people developed metabolic processes that would provide them with the ability to hold out longer during times of famine and be better prepared to live in settled communities.

While some researchers believe that early humans practiced fasting as a way for the community to meet its nutritional needs during times of scarce resources, others believe that early humans first started fasting for religious and spiritual reasons.

Fasting in Ancient Cultures

Ancient Greeks were one of the first civilizations to separate religious fasting from political protest. In ancient Greece, religion, politics and philosophy were all deeply connected in what's known as classical culture.

Until this time, Greeks had observed ritualistic fasting as a way to show reverence to the gods. While these periods of fasting were usually short and not widely practiced, they were important in establishing a connection between the gods and men.

This connection would be an essential part of life for citizens in ancient Greece as each city-state was made up of a multitude of smaller communities, each with its own government and beliefs. The Greek philosopher Plato called this system "democracy" due to people having power over their own lives through their right to vote in civic matters like council members and city officials.

However, this system was not without its flaws. Because the Greek people's beliefs were so diverse, religious leaders often used fasting as a political tool to further their own agenda. Leaders could use periods of either forced or voluntary fasting to coerce people into bending to their will. In his book "The Republic," Plato said:

No human law has ever been able to direct the State aright, and it is but a slight protection for anyone that his commands are obeyed by his own servants and slaves, if there be no higher authority behind them. But for a man to rule and direct his own city, he must be of a noble character, otherwise he will never have any influence.

The prophet Isaiah encouraged fasting more than one thousand years before Christ to show both spiritual devotion as well as political protest. In the Old Testament, Isaiah called on his fellow Hebrews to fast to reject the tyranny they were being subjected to by King Ahaz. Isaiah said "In the day of your fast, you seek your own pleasure, all your workers are idle, yet you do not fast on my behalf." Isaiah prophesized that partaking in fasting and prayer would lead to God's favor and deliverance from King Ahaz's tyranny. This was a continuous source of political protest by leaders who wanted to use fasting as an act of disobedience against the kingdoms they were living under at times of tyranny. In addition to this, many times these same rulers would also claim that their religious beliefs required them to practice fasting.

During the Middle Ages, monks and religious leaders observed fasting as a way to rid their minds of impure thoughts. These periods of spiritual cleansing focused on repentance and communing with God and were tightly regulated under the monastic rules that were in place during this time. Fasting was also used to achieve self-mastery, as the French monk Guigo II mandated in his rule that a monk must have complete mastery of his appetite before he could move on to fasting for any other reason.

CHAPTER 3:

The Myths About Fasting to Dispel

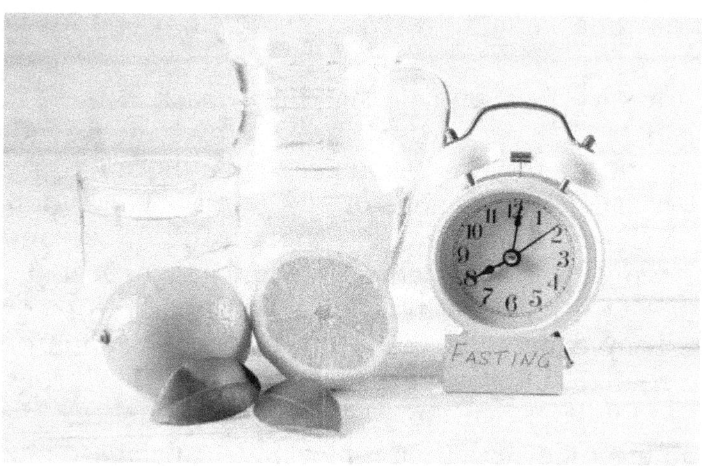

Fasting is an interesting subject to discuss. On the one hand, fasting is so simple—just stop eating food for a certain amount of time. On the other hand, there are many myths and misunderstandings about this seemingly simple act of abstaining from something we all do every day.

Fasting foods and fasting diets are a huge industry. It seems like every few years, some new "fasting" diet shows up on the scene, promising quick and easy weight loss and better health, all without having to give up your favorite foods. Inevitably, many people try it (the diet fad), but most end up quitting because of lack of results or problems with compliance. There are currently fads for a 5-day water fast, a 7-day fast, a 14-day fast etc. It is not uncommon for health seekers to try multiple different fasting regimens before they get one that sticks or before they decide that fasting is just not for them. And that's a shame because fasting, done properly, is one of the most powerful interventions to improve and enhance health.

Misconception #1: Long-Term Fasts Are Dangerous

There is a belief that long-term (24 hours or longer) fasts can be dangerous because they can put your body into starvation mode or increase stress hormones like cortisol. The theory goes that if you do not eat enough, your body will think it's starving and start storing fat for future use. It will also release stress hormones, including cortisol, to help preserve and store energy.

There are very few studies that have tracked the effects of prolonged fasting on cortisol levels. However, a study from Israel in 2015 followed 100 participants over a 24-day Ramadan fast (the longest one studied). They found that fasting for Ramadan had "no significant effect on serum cortisol concentrations", which is what they expected "due to the body's well-known physiological response" to short-term fasting. They concluded that "physiological adaptations may prevent changes in basal cortisol concentrations during longer periods of food deprivation.

Human physiology carries a remarkable capacity to adapt and adjust to extremes of food availability. In the case of prolonged fasting, the body makes adjustments to preserve vital functions while still allowing vital processes to continue uninterrupted. As mentioned earlier, cortisol is one way that your body does this. Another way is by slowing down your metabolism by about 15% during a fast. Your metabolic rate decreases because there are fewer nutrients being pushed through your system. This is why fasting helps you lose fat--it decreases the amount of calories that can be burned by reducing metabolic activity and the number of calories available for burning in the first place. If you give your body enough nutrients to meet its normal metabolic demands, your metabolism will decrease and you'll burn less fat. So, long-term fasting helps you lose fat primarily by decreasing metabolic rate.

Another common myth about fasting is that it puts your body into starvation mode—that is, it halts all non-essential processes and diverts all the remaining energy to vital functions. But it's just not true. During a fast, your body still performs many essential housekeeping activities, such as:

- Storing glycogen (stored carbohydrate) in the liver for use by other organs later.
- Breaking down non-essential fatty acids in adipose tissue (fat stores under the skin) for energy.
- Decreased protein breakdown in muscle.

These are all great ways that your body preserves energy, but it is not a net decrease in metabolic rate. Your body needs to perform all these functions to prevent your physical and mental health from suffering. If you give up fasting because you think it's too dangerous, you may be doing yourself an even bigger disservice.

Misconception #2: Longer Fasts Are Better

Some people believe that fasting longer will yield greater results or more fat loss because the body is "exposed" to starvation for a longer period of time and will respond by increasing metabolic rate, which will help burn more fat. However, nothing could be further from the truth. If you decrease your metabolic rate, it doesn't matter how long your fast lasts, you will lose the same amount of fat. The longer the fast, the more fat loss is slowed. A 24-hour fast decreases energy expenditure by about 5%. A 48-hour decrease is about 10%. A 72-hour decrease is about 15%. And so on. The goal of a proper fasting protocol is not to increase metabolic rate and burn more calories. Rather, the goal is to minimize metabolic activity while maximizing nutrient partitioning—that is, to put nutrients into storage so they are not burned for fuel—so that you have fewer total calories being used in the body over time.

Misconception #3: Fasting Is Not Sustainable Long-Term

Another common misunderstanding about fasting is that people think it must be done only on a short-term basis. The reason for this is that there is a pervasive belief that if you fast for too long, your body will depend on the calories in food and you'll never be able to keep weight off. For example, by reducing calorie consumption by 20% every day for one week, someone with a 2000 calorie per day diet would effectively consume only 1600 calories per day for all seven days of the week—or 800 calories less than their normal 2000 daily calorie diet.

If you were to do this for 30 days, you would have consumed a total of 240,000 calories—or 15,000 fewer calories than your body needs to maintain your current weight. The idea is that if you eat this way for too long, your metabolism will slow or stop and you'll put all the weight back on that you lost. But it's just not true. First of all, a person who starts with a 2000 calorie per day diet will not continue to lose weight if they cut their daily caloric intake by 800 calories every day for 30 days. If you start with 2000 calories per day, your body will try to stay at 2000 calories per day because it's not getting any food. And if you eat only 800 calories per day for 30 days... well, you get the point. In both cases, your body will nearly stop losing weight or even start gaining some weight back.

But let's say that you continue to lose weight despite cutting your daily caloric intake by 800-1000 every day for 30 days. Let's say that by the end of the month, you're eating only 1000 calories per day and still losing 1 pound of fat a week—but now you're only at 1500 calories per day. Will you gain back all the weight you lost?

No. You'll probably gain back some of it because your metabolic rate is still much lower than when you started, and you're using up fewer calories than before. However, what will probably happen is that your metabolism will stabilize at a lower point and use up fewer calories than it did when you started out—perhaps around 1500 calories per day. And this new metabolic rate is much more sustainable long-term.

To recap: to lose weight (and fat), do less damage to your body by eating less food. If you eat less food and still have a lower metabolism than you had when you started, your body will find a new equilibrium point that's not as active as it was before. In other words, it will burn fewer calories and you'll probably gain back some of the weight that you lost—but only if your metabolism is slower than it was before (which usually isn't the case).

CHAPTER 4:

The Benefits of Fasting for Women Over 50

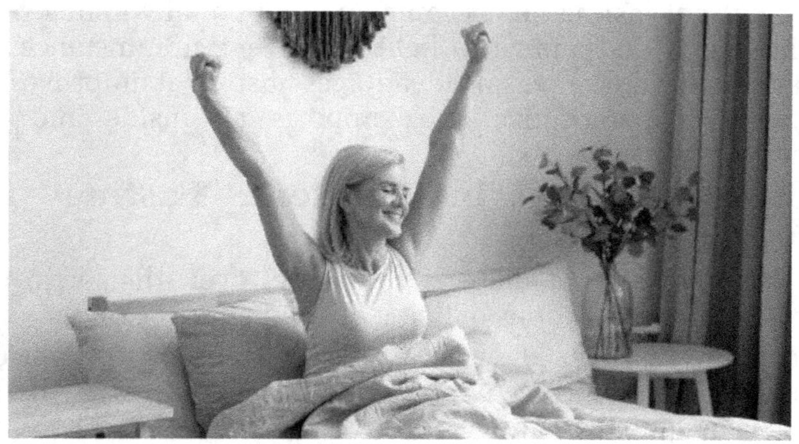

Studies have shown that intermittent fasting might be incredibly helpful for postmenopausal ladies to help in keeping up their weight. There are many advantages to intermittent fasting for moderately aged ladies or ladies who are experiencing menopause regardless of their age.

Why for Women Over 50?

Ladies who approach post-menopause (and in some cases even as right on time as pre-menopause) will, in general, begin to pick up paunch fat. They will begin seeing their digestion get slower. They may likewise begin feeling a throbbing painfulness in their joints. Their rest patterns begin to get totally out of routine, leaving them feeling depleted constantly. At that point, besides the weight acquired, there is a higher danger of creating constant sicknesses like malignancy, diabetes, and coronary illness that could prompt respiratory failures.

Additionally, they face the danger of neurodegenerative illnesses, stroke, and a steady sensation of weakness. Intermittent fasting has been known to reset an individual's inside equilibrium. This, thus, helps their outside appearance, energy levels and eliminates pressure as they control their weight.

For What Reason Should Women Choose the Intermittent Fasting Diet?

Intermittent fasting has become an exceptionally mainstream solid way of life pattern in light of current circumstances. It offers numerous medical advantages just as it improves an individual's perspective and supports an inside and out sensation of prosperity.

Advantages of Intermittent Fasting for Women Over 50

At the point when ladies get to 50 and over, their skin will begin to give indications of being old enough.

They may discover their joints begin to throb for reasons unknown, and unexpectedly tummy fat aggregates as though you have quite recently conceived an offspring. There are countless creams, diets and activities available to fix the skin and attempt to help. The truth of the matter is, they may work in a limited way, then the body hits a rack, and nothing appears to push an individual past it. This bubbles up disappointment, making ladies investigate the more extraordinary and pricey choices, like a medical procedure, which, in itself, presents countless more threats and dangers for ladies of 50 and over.

An individual doesn't have to go under the blade or starve themselves to reboot their framework or change their shape. Intermittent fasting is a lot less expensive and safer approach to do this, and there is no compelling reason to make any radical eating propensity changes by the same token. Indeed, you may have to make a couple of changes like removing shoddy nourishment and eating better. Be that as it may, by and by the diet an individual follows is their own decision and relies upon how genuine they are tied in with getting better.

Some medical advantages of intermittent fasting for ladies over 50 include:

Activating Cellular Repair

Fasting has been known to launch the body's normal cell fix work, dispose of developing cells, improve both life span and chemical capacity. As individuals age many things will generally be regarded as a battering. IF can mitigate joint, muscle and lower back pain. As the cells and any other damage are being fixed, IF assists with the skin's versatility and well-being in general.

Increments Cognitive Function and Protects the Brain from Damage

Intermittent fasting may build the levels of a mind chemical known as a brain-derived neurotrophic factor (BDNF). It might similarly monitor the brain against harm like a stroke or Alzheimer's illness as it advances new nerve cell development. It additionally increments intellectual capacity and could adequately shield an individual against other neurodegenerative ailments also.

Weight Reduction

When individuals have stomach fat, it can cause numerous medical conditions related to different illnesses as it is demonstrated by an individual possessing instinctive fat.

Instinctive fat will be fat that dives deep into the stomach encompassing the organs.

Midsection fat is horribly difficult to lose, particularly for a maturing lady. Intermittent fasting has been known to help diminish weight as well as crawls of over five percent of muscle to fat ratio in around 22 to 25 weeks (Barna, 2019).

Reduces Oxidative Stress and Inflammation

Oxidative pressure is the point at which the body has an irregularity of cell reinforcements just like free radical. This awkwardness can cause both tissue and cell harm in overweight maturing individuals. It can likewise prompt different constant ailments like malignancy, coronary illness, diabetes, and furthermore affects the signs of aging. Oxidative pressure can trigger the irritation that causes these illnesses.

Intermittent fasting can give your framework a reboot, assisting with lightening oxidative pressure and irritation in a moderately aged lady. It likewise altogether decreases the danger of oxidative pressure and irritation for anyone overweight or stout.

Hinder the Aging Process

As intermittent fasting gives both the digestion and cell fix a reboot, it offers the possibility to hinder maturing. It might even draw out an individual's life expectancy by a significant number of years.

CHAPTER 5:

Fasting to Lose Weight

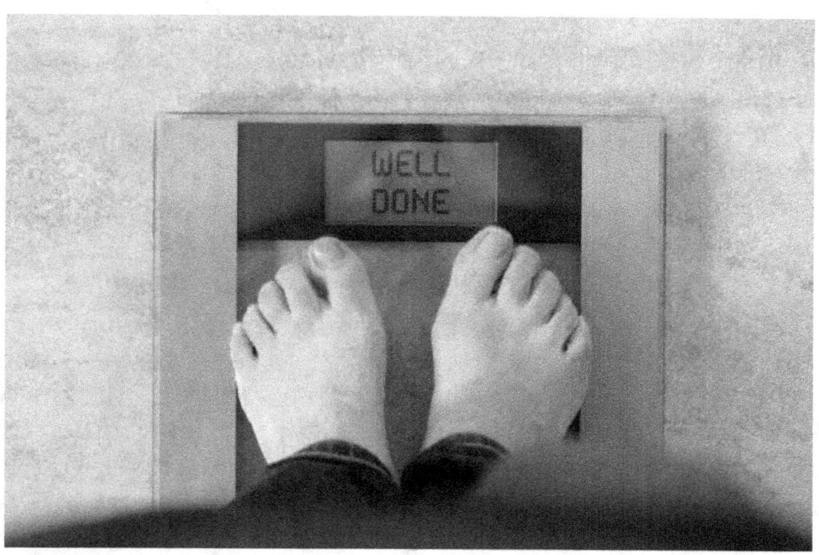

You know that feeling when you're so hungry that you just want to dig your teeth into a burger right here and now? If we could give you a way to reduce those feelings, we reckon that would be pretty great. And as luck would have it—believe it or not—there are such things as intermittent fasting diets!

There are many various types of intermittent fasting diets, but some people also call them "intermittent calorie restriction diets". The idea is that you can reap the benefits of calorie restriction without actually having to count calories for the entire day.

Research has shown some amazing findings on the effects of intermittent fasting for weight loss.

How Does It Work?

In intermittent fasting, you basically commit to eating only during a certain time window and fasting the rest of the day. The most common way is what people call the 16:8 diet, which means you only eat during an 8-hour window. You fast for 16 hours in between. This means that you can eat your first meal at noon and the last one at 8 pm. That's 16/8 or 2am to 10pm on a 24-hour clock.

The magic happens when you're fasting — not because of not eating, but because your body is forced to find alternative ways to fuel itself...

Being active and exercising can actually cause you to burn more calories than you normally would. Plus, your body will tend to crave fewer calories when it has been fasting.

Fasting Is Not Similar to Starving Yourself

One thing to note is that intermittent fasting isn't synonymous with starving yourself. It's simply an alternative way of looking at food intake. When it comes to skin to skin, we always recommend eating for the right reasons, rather than just shoving whatever down your throat whenever you feel like it. That's what leads to binge eating and a big fat mess on the bathroom floor later on.

Intermittent fasting aims at helping you break bad eating habits and get your body into better shape in preparation for weight loss—not the other way around. You'll still be getting all the important nutrients without putting your body into a short-term "survival mode". Everybody wins!

One of the fundamental focal points of intermittent fasting is the possibility to reestablish fat consumption and help the pounds tumble off. Intermittent fasting is preferred over numerous different diets since you don't have to follow your calories by any means, thus you don't have to gauge by any stretch of the imagination. IF prompts expanded fat consumption and quickened weight loss by pushing the body to utilize fat stores as fuel. The body uses glucose as the main source of energy after you eat food. The leftover glucose is put away by the liver and muscle as glycogen.

On the off chance that the body doesn't get glucose, it will utilize its stores to give energy to the body, since numerous cycles going on in the body requires glucose. At the point when you are in a consistent period of fasting, the body will utilize the entirety of the glycogen, and glycogen gets depleted. The body begins searching for different sources to adapt up to the energy interest. Different sources incorporate fat cells, which are broken down to give the energy. This kind of fasting is like a keto diet where the body refuses carbs, and the body utilizes fat to fuel up the body.

CHAPTER 6:

Fasting to Fight Type 2 Diabetes

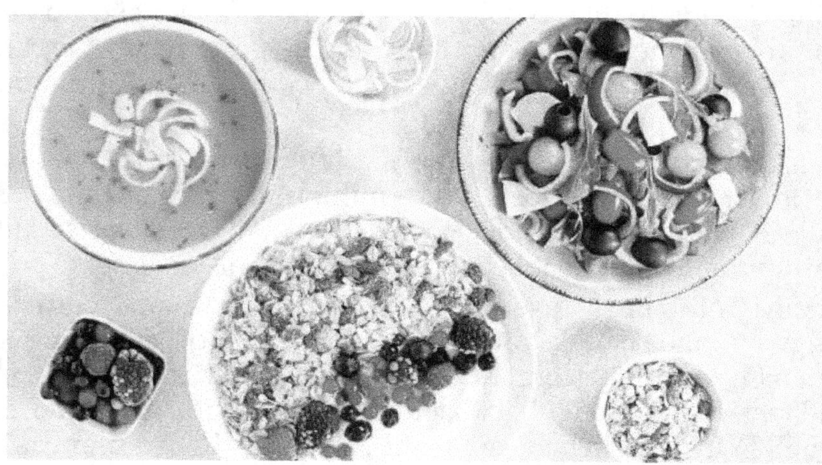

Fasting is a potent instrument for autophagy promotion. Multiple cycles of fasting reduce the burden of metabolites in cells, which leads to improved cell function and protection against some oxidative stressors.

The long-term benefits of fasting are many and range from increased physical stamina, more mental clarity, weight loss—including weight loss from the stubborn fat stores—lower blood pressure and cholesterol levels. Fasting also boosts your immune system and decreases your risk of cancer. New research suggests that not only does it keep you healthier as you age—but it may help ward off type 2 diabetes as well. A study recently published in the journal Cell Metabolism reveals that when mice fast for a 48-hour period, they lose weight, their bodies burn off fat stores and reduce inflammation.

Perhaps more striking is the fact that the mice who underwent this fasting regimen for three consecutive days a week over a six-week period became resistant to type 2 diabetes. They were protected from adult-onset diabetes. Researchers explained that fasting reduced weight gain in obese mice and slowed down aging signs as well, including memory loss and "declining running performance." The calorie restriction also increased muscle mass in rodents, which provided them with more glucose tolerance and insulin sensitivity.

While fasting for three days at a time may be too extreme for you to consider—or even think about—researchers suggest that even two days of fasting can help ward off inflammation and type 2 diabetes.

You know that type 2 diabetes is a huge issue in the western world. It actually affects 25.8 million Americans and 387 million people worldwide, so it's not really a surprise that fasting can be an effective weapon to fight this disease.

Fasting has been used for centuries in many cultures, religions and belief systems as a means of cleansing or repairing the body from illness or injury. In Western medicine and science, fasting has been researched for its potential benefits in treating ailments like type 2 diabetes or heart disease.

Here's a look at how fasting can help in the fight against type 2 diabetes.

Possible Mechanism of Action for Fasting and Diabetes

Type 2 diabetes or adult-onset diabetes is characterized by a group of symptoms that include high blood glucose levels, increased insulin resistance and relative absence of insulin secretion. It's triggered by years of unhealthy lifestyle consisting of a carbohydrate-rich diet, high triglycerides, high blood pressure and inability to exercise on a regular basis. It's very hard to treat for the reason that it's often associated with obesity, which makes the management even more challenging.

Science has offered some explanations as to how fasting can be beneficial in reducing this disease's symptoms. To explain the effects of fasting, it's necessary to focus on how insulin functions in the body.

Insulin is secreted and released into the bloodstream, where it travels to other tissues. It has evolved as a tool for four main purposes:

1) To suppress glucose production in the liver;

2) To stimulate glycogen synthesis;

3) To suppress gluconeogenesis (production of new glucose by non-liver tissues); and, most importantly, to facilitate glucose transport into muscle and fat cells.

Insulin basically facilitates the transportation of glucose from the blood into tissues. In type 2 diabetics, there is resistance to insulin's effects and this is why there's increased blood glucose levels. Hence, with fasting, the body is forced to use up its glycogen supply, which normally acts as fuel for the brain.

During fasting, insulin levels decrease dramatically and there's a shift towards using free fatty acids as fuel. Also, in a study published in Proceedings of National Academy of Science, researchers noticed that during Ramadan (month-long fasting by Muslims), participants' insulin sensitivity increased relative to their blood glucose and insulin levels after meals (known as postprandial glycemic response).

It's important to understand that fasting has been used as a treatment method for many conditions, including epilepsy and other neurological disorders. This is because depriving the brain of glucose actually helps in reducing seizures or other symptoms.

CHAPTER 7:

Fasting to Rejuvenate Your Mind and Body

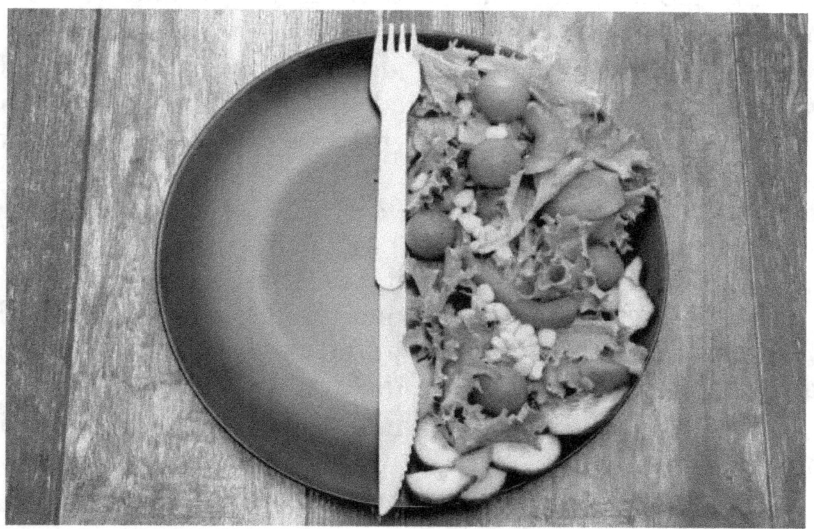

Fasting is the key that unlocks the door to the rest of your health and wellness. It is my opinion that intermittent fasting is one of the most important health breakthroughs in decades. Intermittent Fasting (IF), as it is commonly referred, is simply abstaining from food for certain periods during your day. The periods vary, with some people fasting for 20 hours, while others may fast for 18 hours or more. If you go to sleep by 10:30 at night, you will not be hungry until 2 pm the following day (or later). You can easily go up to 20 hours without eating.

Basically, intermittent fasting involves cycling back and forth between periods of eating and not eating. This can be done daily or on a weekly basis. Intermittent fasting practice can vary from person to person, but typically, a practitioner will simply skip breakfast one day a week; some will also do this on the weekends by skipping breakfast on Saturday and then consuming all calories after 12 p.m.

People who practice intermittent fasting believe that it is a great way to burn fat, boost energy levels, lower blood pressure and improve your overall health. While the jury is still out on intermittent fasting, some doctors agree that it can be a powerful weight-loss tool. That being said, if you're thinking about giving intermittent fasting a shot, here are some things you should know.

Intermittent Fasting has been identified as a popular weight-loss strategy that is practiced by thousands of people. Browsing through articles on the web will show you how people have reported losing significant amounts of weight after switching to an IF diet (intermittent fasting). Surprisingly, there are a lot of young people who are following this type of diet. The majority of these individuals have reported losing up to 10-15 pounds in less than two months. In addition, medical journals and newspapers have also featured this practice as one of the best diets for weight loss.

It has been shown that IF promotes a wide range of benefits. The benefits include:

- Increased energy in the body
- Decreased body fat
- Improved cognitive function
- Improved insulin sensitivity
- Reduced inflammation in the body

Here is some good news for those who are looking to lose weight. Intermittent fasting actually helps you drop pounds, but goes beyond that once you get into a rhythm. It is NOT a diet; it is a lifestyle. I like to think of it as how our ancestors ate before there was food available 24/7. They had periods of time when they may not have eaten for days.

One of the most common misconceptions concerning intermittent fasting is that it is hard to do. In reality, it is very simple. Let's use the example of breakfast. If you are in bed by 10:30 and wake up at 6:30, then a good eating window might be from 12 pm – 12 am, where you would fast for 18 hours. If you drink black coffee or tea in the morning, you don't need to worry about counting that as food towards your eating window.

If you can stick to having your first meal around 12 pm and then eat every three hours after that, you could have a 16 hour fast and an 8-hour eating window.

If you have been trying to lose weight, or if it has been really difficult for you to maintain your weight or even gain, I highly recommend intermittent fasting. It is a lifestyle tool that can help you with more than just losing weight. You could also use this as a way to get started in the morning without eating a high carbohydrate breakfast like oatmeal, yogurt and cereal, etc.

CHAPTER 8:

Fasting to Improve the Cardiovascular System

How can we upgrade the performance of our heart? How can we help it to work more efficiently and be healthier?

As we age, our body starts to deteriorate. And for older people with heart problems, this deterioration is accelerated. The heart is one of the most important organs in our bodies, and its functioning directly affects our health and well-being. It seems that there is no effective way to improve its performance without surgery (open-heart surgery). So, how do we help it work better?

The real secret lies in fasting and observing a proper diet. When followed properly, these diets have proven to give amazing results (even in people suffering from serious illnesses).

The Russian scientist, Dr. Nikolai Anokhin, discovered that in fasting, our heart's activity increases as a result of an increased activity of the parasympathetic nervous systems.

Dr. Anokhin stated: "In the process of fasting, our heart receives a large amount of blood which contains a large amount of oxygen. This results in an important increase in its effectiveness and efficiency".

Fasting is one way to give our body what it needs to keep it healthy and strong, especially when we talk about maintaining an optimal weight and preventing obesity or diabetes.

In a study published in the Journal of Applied Physiology, titled: "Increased sympathetic nervous activity and arterial pressure during fasting", a team of researchers that included Dr. Anokhin found that the activity of our nervous system increases during fasting, especially the activity of our parasympathetic nervous system which relaxes our body and keeps it functioning more efficiently.

The parasympathetic nervous system's increased activity slows down our heart rate, which will help maintain an optimal weight (therefore, preventing obesity or diabetes).

The increased activity will help us to be calmer and more relaxed. That's why experts recommend that patients suffering from insomnia can benefit from fasting.

Scientists have also found that the increased activity in fasting allows a person to have better blood circulation, which helps our heart function more efficiently (since this will help it to receive the required amount of oxygen).

The increased activity will also help our body's organs to work better, and that will improve their performance. This means that fasting might be very important for people with heart problems.

So, how do we know when we should start a fasting period? We can follow these simple rules:

- Our heart should be in a healthy condition or it should have recovered sufficiently after an illness or surgery before we begin fasting.
- Avoid fasting if you have high blood pressure or any other serious illness.
- Fast only if you are healthy and able to continue your normal daily activities.
- Avoid fasting if you are pregnant, breastfeeding or on medication because it may cause negative effects on your health and the performance of your heart.

The benefits of fasting for a healthy heart are amazing: our body will be able to relax, our nervous system will get more active due to the increased amount of oxygen in the blood that reaches our heart. As a result, people with obesity problems or other health problems related to poor blood circulation will benefit greatly from fasting.

So, if you have a healthy heart, then fasting might be a good choice to help it work more efficiently.

Dr. Anokhin's experiments showed remarkable results, even in people with serious illnesses and diseases (cardiovascular problems).

The fasting periods were short (from 5 to 7 days) and medical specialists monitored the subjects.

There are different ways to fast: fruit and vegetable juices (fasting for 5 days), fruit and vegetable juices with honey and yogurt (fasting for 3 days or less), dry fasting (no food whatsoever) under medical supervision. There are different ways of following these diets depending on your needs. So, if you want to help your heart work better and improve your health, you should consider fasting.

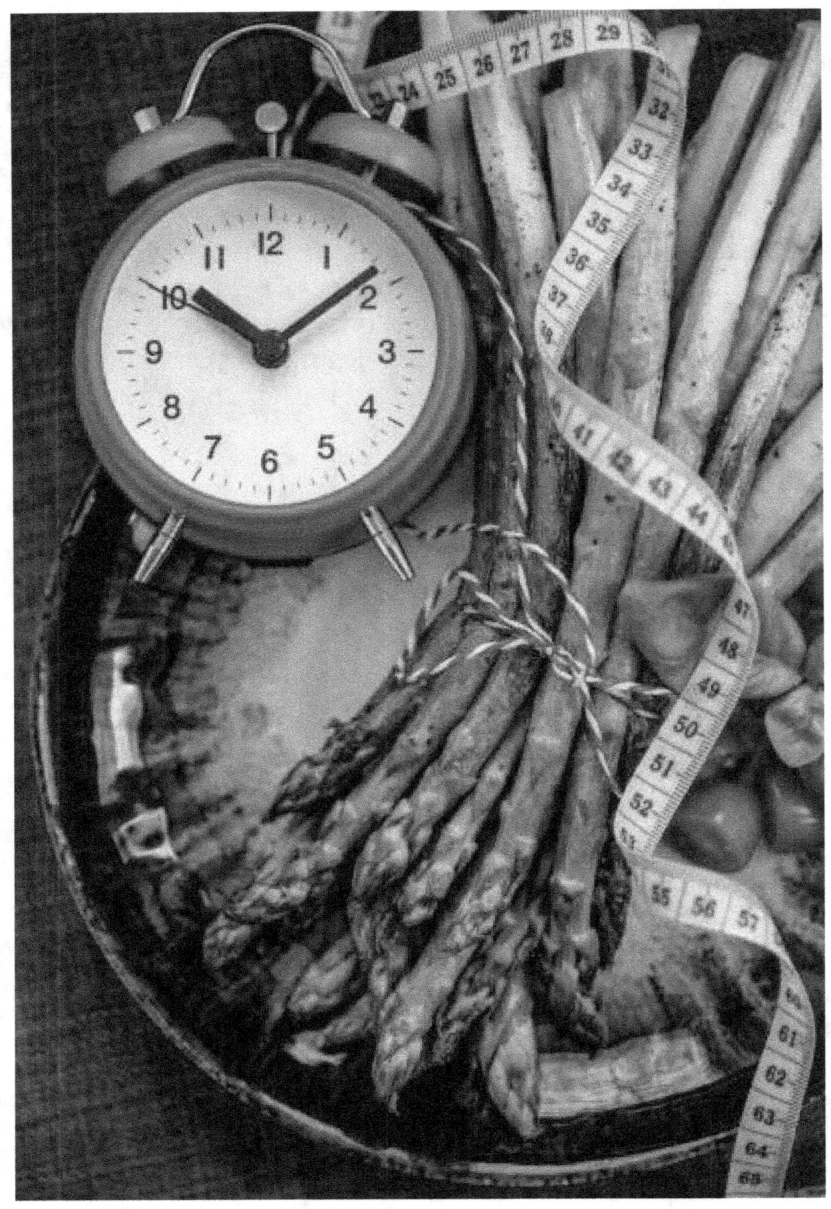

CHAPTER 9:

What You Need to Know About Hunger

If you're fasting, I'm sure you can remember hunger pangs that hit you around the 15-hour mark.

What exactly is this?

Hunger pangs are a primal urge that your body sends you to remind you to eat. It happens when your body "thinks" it's not getting enough nutrients or food to function properly. In fact, hunger pangs don't really last very long...they usually go away by themselves after 15-20 minutes.

Intermittent Fasting is a powerful tool in the fight against obesity. It's a simple way to lose weight without having to count calories.

However, what many don't realize is that the body actually needs food in order to function properly. That's why intermittent fasting is one of the most effective ways to lose weight WITHOUT counting calories!

So, what exactly causes your hunger that you feel after an IF session? A lot of people say it's just because they "forgot" they were supposed to be fasting and ate something else.

But the real reason goes much deeper than that.

Here's what happens...

When you eat, it takes time for your body to process and absorb the nutrients. Then the food will be turned into energy that your body can use. This is true for any meal you take in, whether it's a snack or a 3-course meal.

During this process, two things happen...

(1) You actually feel full! This is because when your body gets enough nutrients, hormones are released to send signals to your brain that make you feel satisfied and full.

(2) Your liver begins breaking down glycogen (a form of sugar stored in the liver) to give your body energy.

If you don't eat, your liver will simply use the glycogen it has stored up to keep your body going. This is basically how you can survive without food for a few days if necessary.

However, there's only so much glycogen in the body. Once this is used up, your body will start using muscle and fat to get the energy it needs from other sources. In fact, lack of food can actually cause fat loss because when you're not eating enough calories on a day-to-day basis, your body will switch to fat burning mode.

As we know by now, our bodies are very good at adapting to our changing circumstances and environments. They change the way we eat; they change our eating pattern; they choose what to burn for energy and so forth.

This is a very good process as it allows us to adapt fast to changes in our immediate environment. However, this makes people feel like hunger pangs are a bad thing. What they forget is that hunger pangs actually serve an important purpose and are part of the natural process of losing weight through IF!

Here's how to conquer your hunger pangs...

1. Make sure you keep consuming enough water throughout the day. Drinks containing caffeine and alcohol will cause dehydration faster.

2. Stay away from high-fat foods. These take longer to digest and can lead to indigestion, acid reflux and stomach problems.

3. Drink a big glass of water before you start your fast. You can drink a glass of water as soon as you finish your fast too! This will help you cut down on the hunger pangs by speeding up digestion giving you more time to burn fat!

4. Eat small meals in between your fasts instead of one big meal. This makes it easier for your body to digest the food slowly, which causes fewer hunger pangs!

5. Get your water requirements from other sources. Drink smoothies and juices instead of plain water during your non-

fasting periods so that you don't realize how much you're actually drinking!

6. Eat some foods which are rich in fiber. These have a slower rate of glycemic index, so they will help you feel fuller for longer!

7. Don't spend too long in between meals, especially in the beginning when you're trying to get used to IF (Learn more about this here). Make sure to get extra protein and water as described above during this time!

8. Don't be too restrictive about your hunger pangs (Learn more about this here). Just because you're fasting all day doesn't mean that you shouldn't have any treats or indulgences. You can still have them—just limit your intake to a small amount!

9. Plan ahead. When you know that you're going to be at work for a long time and there won't be a good time to have your next meal, bring some snacks with you!

10. Get some exercise! This is the best way to burn fat, so make sure to keep it up even when you're doing IF!

CHAPTER 10:

For Whom Fasting Is Not Recommended

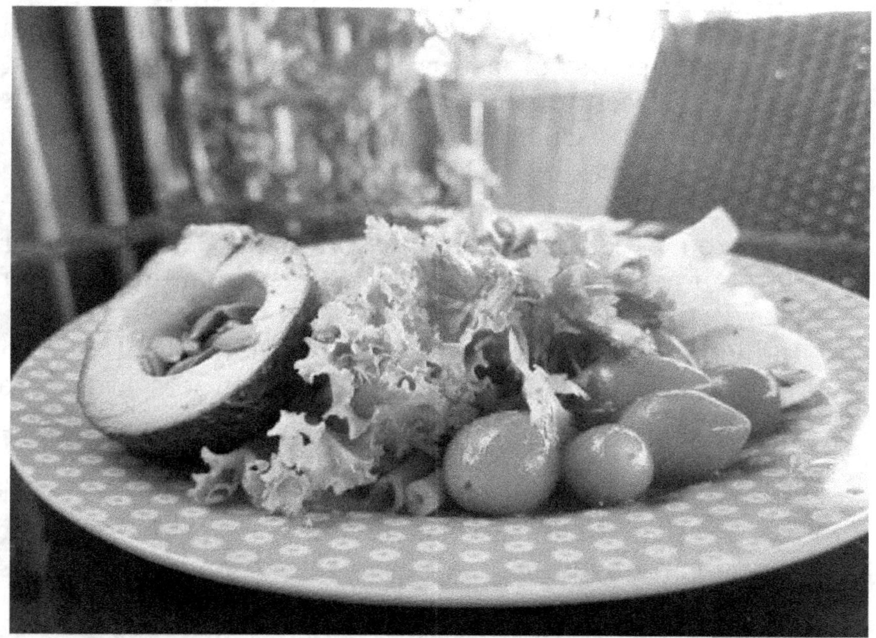

The following type of people should not practice intermittent fasting:

- Diabetics: People with diabetes cannot fast. Fasting puts additional stress on the body, which in turn raises blood sugar and insulin levels. In addition, it is dangerous to deprive diabetics of food since it can increase dehydration and cause hypoglycemia.
- Pregnant Women: Women who are new to intermittent fasting or are considering becoming pregnant should also avoid fasting, as it could result in negative effects on the unborn child.

- People with Low Thyroid Functioning or Undergoing Chemotherapy: Intermittent fasting can inhibit thyroid functioning and lower T3 hormones. It also can interfere with chemotherapy since it lowers the effectiveness of radiation and drug therapy.
- Anyone who is underweight or extremely thin can have difficulty handling intermittent fasting. This is because the body may not have enough stored energy to get through the fast without compromising health.
- The elderly are more likely to suffer from malnutrition after just one day of fasting. Elderly people should eat at least 50 percent of the normal amount of food, which is about 500-600 calories during a 24-hour period.
- Children: According to livestrong.com, children under 12 years old should not practice intermittent fasting. Children require adequate nutrition for proper development, so fasting can be detrimental to their growth process.
- Individuals with other eating disorders: People with anorexia, bulimia, or binge-eating disorders are more susceptible to malnutrition and should not practice fasting.
- People with glycogen storage diseases: People who get easily fatigued after exercising and who feel better after eating carbohydrates may have this disease. Symptoms include hypoglycemia and fatigue after meals.
- People with a family history of diabetes, hypoglycemia or other metabolic problems may be at risk if they fast.
- Obese individuals who are overweight are likely to suffer from low energy levels when fasting. This is especially true when they embark on longer fasts of 1 week or more.
- Individuals with a history of eating disorders such as anorexia or bulimia.

Tips for People Who Are Not Recommended to Practice Intermittent Fasting

- Instead of skipping meals, these people should eat regularly throughout the day. They should also eat more fruits and vegetables to improve digestion and increase energy levels. Meals should be small but frequent.
- People who are newly diagnosed with diabetes should consult a physician before fasting because it could pose risks if done improperly.
- Women who want to get pregnant in the near future should avoid fasting, just in case they become pregnant in the meantime.
- People who are overweight and obese should control their weight before they try to fast. They should also eat a lot of vegetables and fruit.
- Individuals with eating disorders, especially anorexia and bulimia, should get treatment for these first before fasting.

In summary, intermittent fasting is not recommended for pregnant women, diabetics, or people suffering from thyroid conditions or undergoing chemotherapy.

It should also be noted that while intermittent fasting can help with weight loss, it is definitely not a magic pill that can cure obesity. It's unnecessary for some people who manage to lose weight by simply exercising more or watching their diet in general.

CHAPTER 11:

Types of Fasting and Best Practices

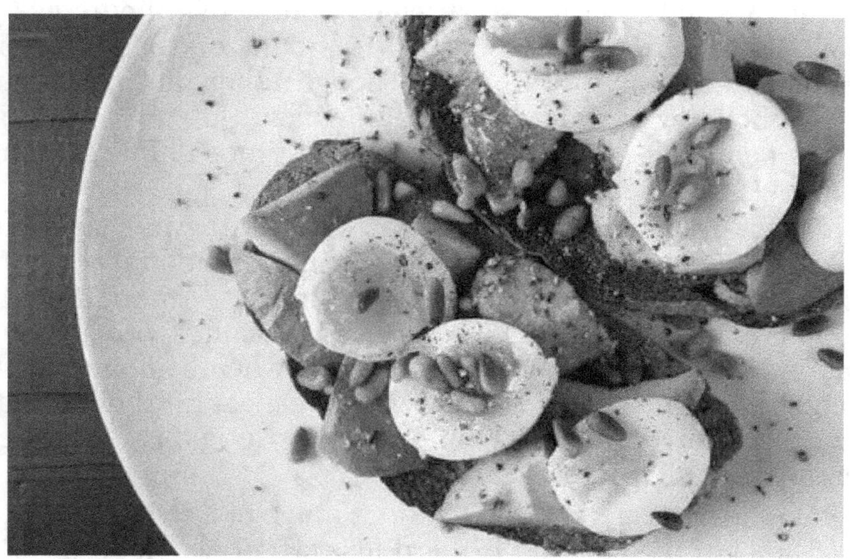

16/8 Intermittent Fasting Method

Quite possibly the most preferred types of fasting for weight loss is the 16/8 intermittent fasting plan. Regularly it's called time-limited fasting; however, a few variations are inconspicuously unique. An individual diets for 16 hours in the 16:8 model and confines the eating to an 8-hour window of time. As a bit of the 16-hour window, a few people miss breakfast. Along these lines, for example, you could eat during the 12 pm to 8 pm range.

However, some people choose to skip dinner regardless. You could confine the eating window to 9 am and 5 pm each day with this. To eat calories, an individual can pick each 8-hour time and miss supper or breakfast.

In any case, you can eat the main feast a day for this fasting pattern. One can pick the circumstance of suppers, similar to breakfast at 10:00 am, lunch will be at 2:00 pm, and supper at 5:30 pm. By 6:00 pm, an individual can wrap up eating their supper, so the entirety of the food utilization is done inside 10 am to 6 pm window, which is eight hours.

As far as possible, the utilization of calorie-containing beverages and food to a restricted window of 8 hours every day. For the remainder of the 16 hours of every day, it includes abstaining from food. Though other diet plans can set unbending standards and guidelines, the 16/8 cycle is more adaptable and dependent on the time-confined taking care of (TRF) method.

This fasting model may assist one with getting in shape and lower the circulatory strain by restricting the amount of hours that one can eat for the duration of the day. An audit study found that the 16/8 procedure assisted lessening with bodying fat and kept up bulk in a few members when combined with actual exercise. A considerably later investigation showed that the 16/8 method didn't impede muscle gains in ladies performing high-impact workout.

While the 16/8 method can, without much of a stretch, fit into each way of life, it could be hard for certain people to try not to eat 16 hours in a row. Also, the potential advantages related with 16/8 intermittent fasting can be totally lost by eating lousy nourishment or such a large number of snacks during the 8-hour window.

To boost this intermittent fasting's medical advantages, try to eat a sound, adjusted diet containing new vegetables, organic products, entire grains, great lean protein, and solid fats.

The 5:2-Method of Intermittent Fasting

The 5:2 diet typically involves devouring ordinary measures of calories to five days every week while lessening your calorie utilization for just 2 days of the week to 500-600 calories. Otherwise called the Fast Diet, was promoted by a British columnists. The 5:2 diet is a basic and direct intermittent fasting plan. You ordinarily eat 5 days every week and don't restrict your calories, but you also don't eat seared or unfortunate bites. At that point, you drop the calorie utilization to one-fourth of your standard necessities for the leftover two days of the very week. This implies decreasing the calorie admission to only 500 calories every day, 2 days of the week, for somebody who routinely burns-through 2,000 calories every day.

As indicated by research, for individuals with type 2 diabetes, the 5:2 diet is just about as proficient as day by day calorie decrease for weight loss and glucose control.

Another examination showed that the 5:2 diet for both weight decrease and the treatment of metabolic problems, for example, cardiovascular disappointment and diabetes, was nearly pretty much as effective as consistent calorie limitation.

As the individual will choose the days they are fasting, the 5:2 diet guarantees adaptability, and there are no rules on whether or what to devour on non-light days. Having said that, it ought to be recalled that eating "for the most part" on non-light days doesn't allow you a free pass to burn-through anything you need.

Alternate-Day Intermittent Fasting

As the title proposes, alternate-day, substitute day intermittent fasting is the point at which one fast or seriously restricts their caloric admission. For substitute day fasting, an individual diets alternate-day. The elective fasting method alternate-day is considerably less mainstream. Moreover, attempting it is maybe the most troublesome type of intermittent fasting. This fasting routine may not be possible. According to the audit study, it might prompt extreme yearning on the fasting days. This other investigation uncovered that the vast majority who could do intermittent fasting were the respondents who attempted to do elective day fasting with an end goal to get in shape. It likewise didn't create greater weight loss or upkeep of weight. Typically, this intermittent fasting isn't unequivocally suggested. For the entire day, it is troublesome not to eat. The individual should stress over their glucose, levels of insulin, and energy.

Your capacity to think can likewise be upset. You will be very ravenous.

An educator of sustenance advocated this methodology. This fast reduced to 25 % of a person's calorie needs, right around 500 calories, on non-fasting. Individuals could fast every other day. This is a typical way to deal with weight loss. In actuality, elective day fasting has been believed to help hefty individuals who need to lose inordinate weight. By about fourteen days, the unfriendly impacts (like extraordinary appetite) reduced, and by about a month, the members kept on getting more comfortable with the diet. The downside was that, during the two months test, respondents said they never truly felt their stomachs were full, which can make it hard to stick to this fasting method.

24-Hour fast/ One Meal a Day

Between dinners, try to fast for 24 hours. Eat at 7 pm right off the bat, for instance, and fast until 7 pm the next day. On the other hand, an individual can decide to eat prior, either lunch or breakfast and fast until the following day for 24 hours. The idea is that consistently you eat a feast yet permitting your body to fast for a more extended timeframe. Such a fasting is normally performed more than once per week; however, it very well may be all the more regularly received. This sort of fasting isn't for everybody.

The OMAD intermittent fasting (one supper daily) is the point at which one restricts our eating window to just a single hour out of each day, and for the leftover 23 hours, fasting occurs. This is a definitive kind of intermittent fasting, and for some people, it very well may be a compelling methodology for extraordinary weight loss.

Eat-Stop-Eat

Eat Stop Eat is an unconventional way to deal with intermittent fasting advocated by an "Eat Stop Eat" columnist. This intermittent fasting plan incorporates characterizing a couple of non-back-to-back days every week for a 24-hour cycle during which one avoids eating or fasting. One can eat unreservedly during the remaining days of the week, however, it is recommended to eat a balanced diet and stay away from excessive consumption.

The purpose for a 24-hour fast consistently is that eating fewer calories will at last prompt weight loss. Fasting for 24 hours can bring about a metabolic move that makes one's body use reserve fat instead of glucose as a fuel source. In any case, it requires a gigantic measure of self-restraint to evade nourishment for 24 a ridiculous amount of time and may prompt gorging later on. It might likewise bring about eating disorder patterns.

The Warrior Diet

This intermittent fasting plan is known as the champion diet, dependent on old fighters' eating patterns. The Warrior Diet, which was created in 2001, is somewhat more sensational than the 16:8 methods yet less inflexible than Eat Stop Eats' method. It consists of eating basically nothing or almost nothing during the day for 20 hours; then eating as much food as wanted around evening time in a 4-hour window. During the 20-hour fast period, the Warrior Diet elevates individuals to devour little amounts of hard-bubbled eggs, dairy items, vegetables, and crude leafy foods without any calories. After the 20-hour fast, in a 4-hour eating window, people can eat anything they need, however, it should be natural. Natural nourishments and solid are proposed. Despite the fact that there is no research, particularly on the Warrior Diet, it considers that time-limited feeding cycles can boost weight loss.

There could be numerous other well-being favorable circumstances of time-limited taking care of periods. Studies demonstrate that taking care of cycles that are time-confined can hinder diabetes, limit tumors' advancement, defer aging, and improve life expectancy. More examination on the Warrior Diet is expected to get a handle on its weight-loss preferences completely.

Spontaneous Meal Skipping

To appreciate any of its focal points, you don't have to embrace a formal intermittent fasting plan. Another decision is to miss dinners from time to time, for example, cooking and eat and not devouring when you are excessively occupied or don't feel hungry. It's a confusion that individuals should burn-through calories before they enter hunger mode or lose their muscles like clockwork. Your body is decidedly ready to adapt to protracted stretches of appetite, not to mention the loss of one to two dinners every now and then.

Subsequently, one day you simply don't feel hungry, miss breakfast, and just have a decent lunch or supper. Or then again, in case you're going anyplace and you can't discover something you need to devour, do it effectively and immediately. It's basically an irregular inconsistent snappy to miss a couple of dinners whenever you are enticed to do as such. Just ensure during different suppers to burn-through nutritious nourishments.

Choose-Your-Day Fasting

This is a greater amount of an experience willingly. Each and every other day or on more than one occasion every week, you could do time-limited fasting as you fast for 16 hours, and to eat for eight hours implies that Saturday could be an ordinary eating day, and by 8 p.m. one would quit eating; at that point, around early afternoon on Sunday, the eating will be continued. It resembles skipping breakfast a few days per week.

3.9 Time-Restricted Fasting

With this type of intermittent fasting, a constant window of care is chosen, which will preferably leave a 14 to 16-hour fasting window. It is prescribed for ladies over 50 to fast for close to 14 hours every day because of hormonal issues. Fasting supports autophagy, the basic and solid cell housekeeping measure in which the body clears declined protein, cell flotsam and jetsam, and different things that impede the method of mitochondrial well-being, which starts when the body's glycogen is drained, specialists say. Doing it could help expand the digestion of fat cells and help improve the capacity of insulin.

For everything to fall into place, an individual may set their eating window from 9 a.m. To 5 p.m. This can function admirably for someone with a family who is as yet eating an early supper. Decidedly a lot of the time invested in fasting is still energy spent snoozing. Contingent upon that, when an individual sets their eating window, you will not miss any suppers. Yet, this relies upon how predictable one can be. In the event that your timetable is entirely adaptable, or you need the opportunity to go out sometimes for breakfast, or you need delayed suppers, it may not be for you to have day-by-day fasting cycles.

CHAPTER 12:

Intermittent Fasting

What is Intermittent Fasting?

Intermittent Fasting (IF) is the act of fasting for a specific period, then eating for another predetermined timeframe and going through this process repeatedly. As the name states, you are fasting intermittently. These fasting and eating times can fluctuate, however, they are generally somewhere near twelve hours of each, cycled each day. Different instances of intermittent fasting systems could be fasting for 16 hours in a day and afterward an eating window of 8 hours. As a rule, when you practice IF, you will isolate your day or your week into eating and fasting areas of time, which will repeat either consistently or consistently. With this kind of fasting, you can ingest fluids with zero calories like water, espresso, tea, in any event, during times of fasting. Simply be certain that adding sugar to your espresso or dark tea will break your fast.

How Can It Work?

Intermittent fasting is getting progressively famous for losing fat, conditioning, and improving well-being. In any case, what are the standards behind this methodology, and what are the focal points? Fasting consistently signifies "without food." This can go from a couple of hours (think rest, for instance) to a couple of days. While a few projects depend on at least one 24-hour fasts each week, this isn't the best way to accomplish fasting. One of the genuine preferences of this diet over other potential diets is that it can adjust to your life. In the event that a 24-hour cycle suits you, great, if not, a 16 or 20-hour time frame may work better.

Does fasting imply that nothing can be consumed? The appropriate response here is no and very the inverse. The upside of fasting is that it can "reset" your body to purge itself.

This is troublesome if the stomach-related plot is forever troubled by steady assimilation. Drinking more water and green tea during this time can help and accelerate the purging cycle. Maybe the most thought little part of intermittent fasting is its effect on the measure of food we eat. Rather than eating for the duration of the day (a totally unnatural approach to eat), the time frame without food naturally diminishes calorie admission. It not only permits you to feel full with the food you burn, but also improves stomach-related capacity during the fasting windows.

This is quite possibly the main medical advantages IF offers. While we will investigate that in more depth, remember that intermittent fasting is a magnificent fat loss way of life diet, particularly for individuals hoping to get rid of stomach fat, which is connected to coronary failures and other difficult issues.

Some intermittent fasting cycles will break a fast period with 24 hours or an entire day of eating whatever your heart wants. The food comprises of fixings that you would ordinarily devour, similar to dairy items, fats, and carbs. However long you return to a fasting period the following day, your body and digestion can figure out how to consume rather than store food and have sufficient time between each huge dinner to appropriately process your food. This is only one of the numerous arrangements that take into consideration days where you eat typically. This recurrent intermittent fasting diet can be appealing to individuals who like to eat or when you have significant get-togethers that you would prefer not to miss that incorporate heaps of eating.

The main motivation behind why you ought to think about this diet is that it is a demonstrated method of shedding pounds without adding additional weight on your body.

The fast days permit our digestion to work pretty hectically as there is enough to consume in our body because of the past "eating" day! Interestingly, the digestion doesn't back off on the grounds that "it knows" that we are taking care of it one more day, and the cycle is repeated, which just causes us to consume calories faster; an ideal and solid arrangement.

Numerous individuals are starting to see the connection between fasting and weight loss and are encountering all the advantages of sound and characteristic weight loss. Intermittent fasting is even said to help you live longer since it improves insulin resistance condition, which is the biggest factor for some well-being factors, including weight loss and muscle building, against aging, and infection avoidance.

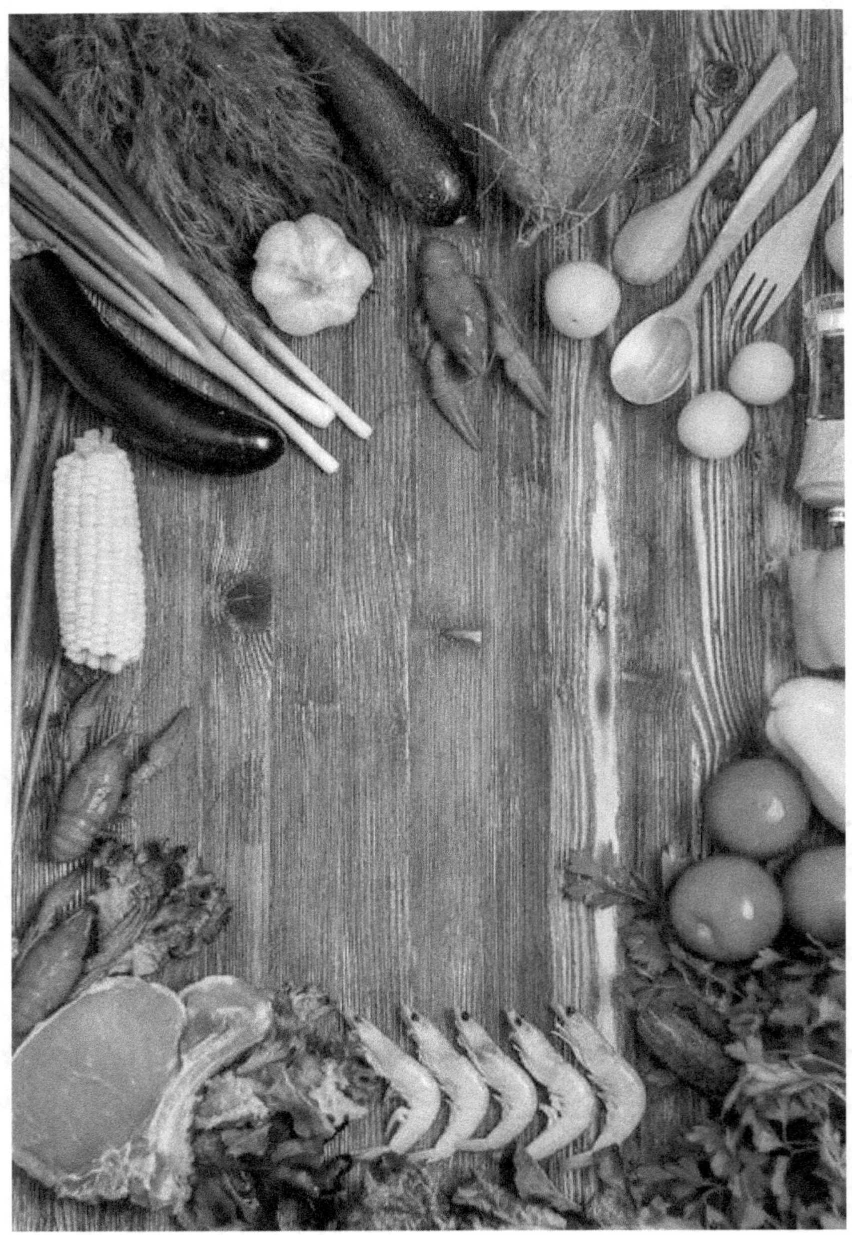

CHAPTER 13:

Longer-lasting Fasts (24-42 hours)

24 Hour Water Fasting

Water fasting is a method of fasting where an individual doesn't ingest anything aside from water for a while. Numerous individuals practice water fasting for times of around 24 hours (yet that can be as long as 72 hours). The choice in regards to the length of your water fast should be made with the assistance of a specialist.

On the off chance that you have at any point gone into the emergency clinic for an operation, they probably revealed to you that you were unable to eat food and could just drink water for a specific period before the intervention. This training would have been a type of water fasting. A few people likewise attempt water fasting as a method of "detoxing" their bodies. Another utilization for it, however, is to prompt autophagy physically. Numerous individuals practice times of water fasting to instigate autophagy to free their assortment of possibly hurtful infections or microorganisms with an end goal to diminish their danger of sicknesses, for example, disease and Alzheimer's and even increment their life expectancy. This is a direct result of autophagy's purging properties, as it stalls contaminated cells and utilizes their salvageable parts for new and solid cells to be created. As you probably are aware, from perusing the past part, autophagy can profoundly affect the disease.

Autophagy can lessen the danger of malignant growths because it gets the body free from harmed cells, which could somehow collect and form into disease.

There are added advantages of water fasting that don't straightforwardly include autophagy yet are important in any case. Water fasting has been appeared to diminish pulse, cholesterol and even improve the working of insulin in the body, hence improving glucose.

The issue with water fasting is that it very well may be very hazardous if not rehearsed in a safe and observed manner. Counsel a specialist prior to endeavoring a water fast with the goal that you can guarantee you are doing as such in a protected manner. There are a few gatherings of individuals who ought not practice water fasting. These gatherings incorporate pregnant ladies, kids, the older, and individuals with eating issues.

Something else to remember while endeavoring a water fast with an end goal to shed pounds is that the weight lost during a water fast may not be the specific sort of weight that you are attempting to lose. During a water fast, there is an extreme limitation in calories, which prompts the breakdown of fat stores, however, a portion of the weight you have lost could likewise incorporate water weight, put away starches, and some of the time muscle (in longer fasts). This means after a water fast, the weight you have lost may return rapidly if the larger part was water or sugar stores, as these are renewed rapidly once an individual starts eating once more. If so, don't be concerned, this is an exceptionally typical response for your body to have as it is worked to foresee surprising fasts and subsequently has approaches to shield you from these, for example, putting away carbs.

When moving toward a water fast, it is helpful to set up your body for a couple of days, paving the way to it by tightening your eating rations to eliminate food from your day, bit by bit. This will better set up your body to abandon nourishment for a day or two. Another approach to get your body accustomed to water is to fast for part of the day so it can get acquainted with investing some energy without food. You may likewise be thinking about how a water fast could cause you to lose water weight, yet it is totally conceivable and even likely. This is on the grounds that a large part of the water we bring into our bodies for the duration of the day is encased in the food sources we eat. On the off chance that your water admission stays as before, yet your food ingestion drastically diminishes, you could wind up getting got dried out and hence losing water weight.

You will likewise have to change your exercises to oblige this water fast, particularly in the event that it is your first time attempting it. If you are not used to fasting, you may feel dazed, which may make a portion of your day-by-day undertakings more troublesome. This could be because of lower glucose or lower circulatory strain on the off chance that you are got dried out. Make certain to remember this as you endeavor a water fast, and make certain to build your water admission to keep away from a drop in circulatory strain.

There is still considerably more exploration that should be finished encompassing water fasting in people specifically. Water fasting as a method of weight loss is a moderately new methodology and one that is simply starting to be investigated with human guineas pigs.

Eat-Stop-Eat or The 24-Hour Fast

This method is the most extraordinary method you can discover. It should just be finished by genuinely experienced professionals of the intermittent fasting approach.

Furthermore, you need to develop your endurance to get to this level. For example, a few people get going with a 12/12 methodology, at that point 14/10, 16/8, 18/6, 20/4, and afterward hit the 24-hour mark.

Prior, we referenced that abandoning nourishment for 24 hours can be perilous. This way, you may encounter indications like unsteadiness, weariness, migraines, and on the off chance that you are snared on sugar and carbs, you may encounter withdrawal side effects (peevishness, uneasiness, and even extreme cerebral pains).

Overall, this methodology isn't suggested except if it is done under clinical watch. This is particularly evident on the off chance that you have any sort of ailment. In such cases, it very well may be astute to forego endeavoring this method.

In any case, you should check it out as a method for a test. While there are people who practice this methodology consistently, say double seven days, most experts take part in it generally a few times per month.

Moreover, kindly try to slope down your caloric admission on the day preceding your fast and steadily increase your caloric admission during the following day. Additionally, make a point to keep your actual work moderate. This sort of challenge is best done at home and in the organization of other people who can watch out for you. On the off chance that you endeavor this test, be prepared to have an extremely quick bite, should you feel any of the indications depicted before. For example, leafy foods are a great method to assist you with recovering security.

36-hr Fasting

Fasting for longer than 24 hours is where all the magic begins. The more you say in a fasting state, the more your body is forced to trigger its supply systems that start to draw on fat stores, bolster rejuvenating microorganisms and reuse old wrecked cell material through the system of autophagy. It takes, at any rate, an entire day to see significant signs of autophagy. Yet, you can speed it up by eating low carb before starting the fast, rehearsing on an unfilled stomach, and drinking homemade teas that facilitate the challenge. If you think about it, 36 hours is not that much. You can eat the night before, then fast during the day, go to sleep on an empty stomach, wake up the next day, fast a few more hours, and begin eating again.

You can still drink mineral water, plain coffee, green tea and some types of teas.

CHAPTER 14:

Prolonged Fasts

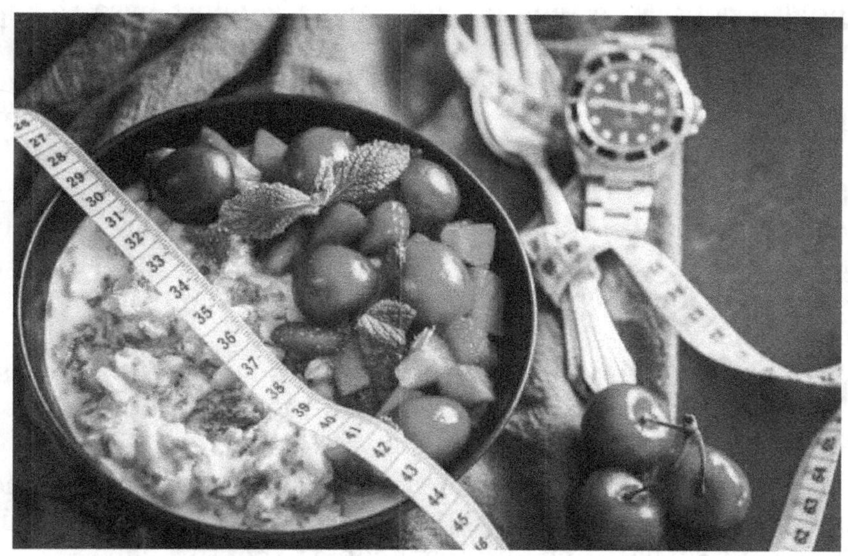

Prolonged fasts are one of the most enticing tools a person can employ in improving health. It takes commitment and discipline to use the powerful tool of a prolonged fast for persons with serious health issues, and it is important to understand how this powerful tool works. In weeks where people eat nothing, they need to be eating high-quality unprocessed foods the days prior to begin and following their prolonged fast with excellent food choices.

Prolonged Fasts are probably among the most challenging things any motivated individual can perform for themselves. It's definitely not an easy way out to lose weight by just not eating. Both a prolonged fast and water fasting are tools of the spirit.

Spiritually, it requires deep inner work; physically, it requires great discipline to leave the physical body intact and provide it with the essential nutrients needed during a fast. It is a core part of the masculine journey to face this challenge at least once in our lifetimes, whether we are male or female.

The other side of this coin is why some choose not to go for long periods without eating. Some cannot get through an initial fast because they do not have a support base set up around them to help them get through those first few days, which can be very challenging. Some of us have been on and off diets our whole lives; we are addicted to food and thus cannot endure a prolonged fast.

However, those of us who are committed to personal growth will experience a transformation in ourselves through the challenges of fasting; it's not easy to do from an ego perspective, but there is a profound spiritual reward for facing that challenge.

It is important to understand how this powerful tool works. The body has three phases it goes through during prolonged fasts.

The first phase, the catabolic state, occurs when there is no food for the body and begins between 3-5 days into a fast. This state is not an easy one for most people to get through.

The body begins to scavenge on its own tissue by breaking down muscle tissues. This is the "breaking down" phase of the fast, where some people experience fatigue, cravings and intense hunger pains; it is during this stage of the fast that many people throw in the towel and start eating food again, only to gain back all of the weight they lost plus some.

However, those who are committed to healing their bodies with fasting as a tool will question why they feel so bad during this stage of fasters and see this as a sign that it's detoxification taking place.

Eating our own fat tissue is the body's main source of energy during this stage. The liver and kidneys begin to clean out the toxins stored in our fat tissue, which is one of the reasons some will experience a drastic weight loss during this stage in their fast.

The catabolic stage may last for 10 days or longer. It also depends on how much toxic material there is to be released from the body and how much energy reserves are left in your body, which will determine how long this may take.

Stage two: Autophagy takes place during autophagy and continues into the beginning of stage three of a prolonged fast.

Autophagy begins to occur when the liver begins to produce ketone bodies, also known as ketosis, which means that the body is beginning to use fat as energy instead of stored sugars in muscle tissue.

If you are going through this stage of a fast and do not feel any cravings at all for food, but feel tired sometimes or experience mild headaches, you may be in Ketosis.

Stage three: Metabolic Change occurs as the body becomes more efficient at using fat reserves for energy. This stage starts 45-90 days into fasting. The body begins to use ketones derived from fat cells for energy instead of tearing down muscle tissue and producing metabolic wastes during catabolism.

This stage is also known as the healing or regenerative stage of a fast, and many people experience a total body transformation during this stage of a prolonged fast.

The ketone diet has been demonstrated to have great benefits in helping to heal cancer tumors. This is because cancer cells do not access energy from ketones, but regular healthy cells do.

It is important for someone fasting to be eating unprocessed high-quality foods lead up to their fast as well as following their prolonged fast with excellent food choices.

CHAPTER 15:

Fasting Tips and Frequently Asked Questions

These tips will assist you with getting acclimated to IF rapidly once you start.

Drink Water

Lack of hydration is something that can wreck you off your way before long. Your body will relinquish any overabundance of water it holds initially and you will see a drop in weight.

Try not to confuse this with fat loss, in any case, it's simply water weight.

Regardless of this water being viewed as superfluous, a particularly abrupt arrival of liquid can trigger a lack of hydration in certain individuals. The activity is to avoid any and all risks and keep it from the beginning. Buy a water bottle that has markings on it, so you realize how much water you're drinking for the duration of the day.

Intend to drink marginally more than your necessary admission level and screen yourself for the side effects of parchedness. Remember that activity will bring about water loss and you ought to recharge this water however much as could be expected.

You may be enticed to imagine that caffeinated beverages will do the work, but recall that they contain a great deal of sugar and aren't the most ideal alternative for you.

Stick to past water and you'll be fine.

Plan Ahead

Take some time the prior night to prepare. When will your fasting window end and can you eat dinner around then? At the point when will you cook and do you need to prepare.

Preparing is something that will generally catch individuals out generally.

In any case, receive a preventive way to deal with all the things you require to do and plan everything out. During the day, attempt to remain dynamic and occupied with assignments.

This will get your brain far from food and appetite. The initial not many occasions you do IF, you will feel hungry.

Remember that this isn't your body feeling hungry. It's essentially a response to it anticipating that food then thanks should the manner in which it has been adapted. At the end of the day, it's clock hunger and isn't genuine. You can attempt to drink some water as of now or have some espresso to push it back. Over the course of seven days, you'll see that your body will conform to it and you'll be fine.

Use Coffee and Tea

At the point when clock hunger strikes your closest companions will be espresso and tea. Tea is a particularly decent decision, explicitly green tea. Green tea is a great source of cell reinforcements and assists battle against free radicals. On top of this, drinking liquids decreases those cravings for food that will happen during the primary week when you're embracing IF.

Join IF with Other Protocols

Whenever you've accustomed to IF, you can probably manage to join it with a low carb diet, for example, the ketogenic diet. This will assist you with losing fat much faster. Remember that the keto diet is certifiably not a simple one to follow, particularly for veggie lovers. The best way to deal with the intake is to slide into it.

You can begin by following it on your rest days to check whether you're ready to make it work. If so, you can grow it to your exercise days. Your body will set aside some effort to change in accordance with the keto diet. Frankly, the actual diet is the subject of a whole book and, in light of a legitimate concern for space, I'll confine myself to a couple of significant focuses.

The main point to remember with keto is that your body will set aside some effort to change from consuming carbs to fat. Take into consideration that carbs are the essential fuel source and your body won't flip a switch and begin consuming fat basically. There is a progress period and this is regularly alluded to as the keto mist.

During this time, which goes on for a week or somewhere near, you will feel less invigorated and you'll feel as though you're not ready to escape second stuff. The haze goes on for a week and once this time passes, your body will actually want to consume fat as its essential source of fuel pretty without any problem. Rehearsing keto on your non-preparing days is a decent method to get your body used to consuming fat as its essential fuel source.

The most ideal approach to get ready for keto is to prepare of time and ensure your dinner prep is on point. Continuously start with your protein admission and afterward move to different macros. It is ideal to figure your macros and calories forthright and afterward keep your suppers as uniform as conceivable to maintain a strategic distance from calorie checking getting overwhelming.

Simplicity yourself into keto much as you would with IF, and you'll see that the two conventions consolidated will have a monstrous effect on your overall wellbeing.

Try Not to Binge

A typical mistake that amateurs make is to see in the start care of the window just like a crazy situation all things considered. From the beginning, this can be difficult to oppose since it will look at the fasting time frame just like a no man's land with no food at all. The explanation this perspective creates is on the basis that people consider IF as prohibitive.

At the point when I say prohibitive, I imply that a few people consider it a convention where you deny yourself nourishment for a while and need to utilize your reserve to prevent yourself from eating. Consider this: Human creatures are all around intended to fast. Consider how our progenitors lived before we created urban areas and cultivates and brought forth the Kardashians.

Food was scant and wasn't ensured. All things considered, there isn't any deer in this world that will readily offer itself up to be eaten. Individuals needed to experience periods where there wasn't any food accessible; they actually figured out how to endure. We've come to connect the clock with our supper times and as a rule, we feel clock hunger and not genuine yearning.

It's arrived at where a few people don't have a clue what yearning feels like. On the off chance that is just bringing you back into your regular eating pattern and is keeping you from going down the bunny opening of permitting the clock to direct what your stomach needs.

No, I'm not making that up! You can see his line of thought. You can't jerk off in case you're pushing horrendous grain into your face, can you? In any case, that is the foundation story of the supposed "most significant feast of the day". There is no confirmation of any unfriendly impacts of skipping breakfast or of not eating breakfast during the time assigned for it.

All things considered, don't stress over skipping breakfast or even a dinner. The only thing that is in any way important is your calories in versus out. Perceive what clock hunger is and get back in contact with your body's necessities.

FAQS

Question # 1: Can I Take Bone Broth?

Above all else: what is bone broth - and for what reason would anybody be keen on taking it?

So, bone broth is the beverage acquired by heating up the bones and connective tissue of various kinds of creatures.

It is plentiful in nutrients, minerals, collagen, and different supplements.

What's more, it is exact in light of the fact that the bone stock is wealthy in supplements that it gets fascinating for longer fasts, since it can supplant supplements (nutrients and minerals) lost during the fasting window.

All things considered, you are often killing water and minerals during this period through pee and sweat.

Question # 2: What Breaks Fasting?

There is no single response to this case—however serenely, we should clarify it appropriately.

What's more, before the end, you will comprehend the reality of why a few people say that a specific food or drink "breaks" fasting and why others say it doesn't.

Indeed, the response to that question is to recognize two sorts of fasting: insulin fasting and calorie fasting.

Question # 3: What Can I Eat or Drink During Fasting?

As we said before, to receive the full rewards that intermittent fasting can give, you basically shouldn't eat or drink whatever has calories.

Then again, we also contend that limited quantities of good fats won't upset your objectives if you are simply hoping to control your insulin.

Lastly, we additionally say that a few authors safeguard the possibility that eating not very many calories (up to 50 kcal) would not break your fast—paying little heed to the source of those calories.

All things being equal, we realize that a few people lean toward a rundown of food sources to assist them with beginning.

This functional rundown helps with remembering which nourishments and beverages can or can't be burned-through during the fast window - without fundamentally "breaking your fast" or finishing every one of its advantages.

Question # 4: But shouldn't something be said about Sweetened Foods But No Calories? Like Coffee with Stevia, Erythritol or Sucralose, and even Zero Soda?

At this point, you have perceived that the possibility of intermittent fasting isn't to burn-through food—so as not to ingest calories or to raise insulin.

Anyway, utilizing non-caloric sugars would be delivered, correct?

Quiet down—this issue is more perplexing than it might appear from the start.

To begin with, I firmly suggest that you understand the contrasts between the various sorts of low-carb sugars.

However, as we clarified, regardless of whether we consider just sugars that don't raise insulin (similar to the case with stevia, or even erythritol, for instance), we actually have a significant inquiry.

That (albeit this relationship is speculative—that is, dubious), there are conceivably a few possible instruments through which the utilization of sugars can meddle with digestion.

Also, that even incorporates collaborations with sweet taste receptors, which would invigorate other metabolic transformations.

Positively, more examination is required, however, as we would like to think, this is one more sign that it very well may be savvy not to mishandle sugars.

Question # 5: Intermittent Fasting Causes Loss of Muscle Mass (Lean Mass)?

Another exceptionally normal inquiry is with respect to the preservation of bulk when we work on fasting.

This inquiry emerges for the most part since we generally hear around (particularly repeated as a mantra in exercise centers) that on the off chance that you didn't eat like clockwork, your body would begin to consume muscles to give you energy.

Unfortunately, this is a typical legend—and we simply have no clue about where it came from.

In the event that you read the inquiry concerning "eating like clockwork" that we replied above, at that point you understand that you don't need to eat at regular intervals to ration your bulk.

Then again, you might be contemplating whether taking longer periods without eating (16, 24, 48 hours or more) would harm your lean mass.

However, you can sit back and relax: you won't break muscles as a type of energy during the fasting window.

CHAPTER 16:

Drinks Compatible with Fasting

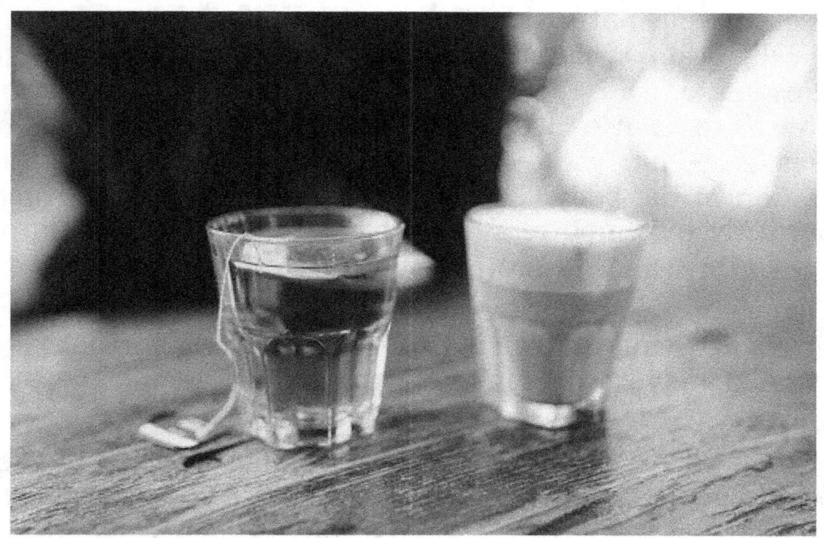

With the most recent diet upset, intermittent fasting has gotten amazingly mainstream and it is said that this can likewise help get thinner faster. Numerous individuals, particularly youngsters, follow a controlled fasting plan—going on a long time of no-eating and afterward eating once more. Yet, what to eat when you do eat?

The main thing to remember is that you don't need to go overboard on calories when you do eat. Try not to top off on bunches of extra carbs.

Few Beverages That Are Viable with IF

Water

Plain or carbonated water contains no calories and will keep you hydrated during a fast. Water is consistently a decent decision. This will likewise help keep your stomach full while keeping a negligible carbohydrate level. At the point when you are fasting, it is essential to likewise keep up legitimate hydration levels.

Espresso and Tea

Most of these should be consumed without added sugar, milk or cream. However, some people find that adding modest amounts of milk or fat can control hunger.

Green tea has anti-oxidant properties and is known to help your digestion. It has a large portion of the caffeine of dark tea or espresso, and therefore, doesn't influence your dozing patterns or pulse like espresso can. It likewise contains epigallocatechin gallate, which represses prostaglandin E2 creation in the body. This forestalls aggravation all through your body and empowers solid weight loss around the midriff.

Diluted Apple Juice Vinegar

A few people find that drinking 1–2 teaspoons (5–10 ml) of apple juice vinegar blended into water can help them stay hydrated and forestall longings during a fast.

Sound Fats

A few people drink espresso containing MCT oil, ghee, coconut oil, or spread during their fast. Oil breaks a fast, yet it will not break ketosis and can hold you over between dinners.

Bone Stock

This rich wellspring of supplements can help renew electrolytes lost during extensive stretches of just drinking water.

Smoothies

Mixed beverages can be a gentler method to acquaint supplements with your body since they contain less fiber than entire, crude leafy foods.

Soups

Soups containing protein and effectively absorbable carbs, such as lentils, tofu, or pasta, can tenderly break a fast. Evade soups made with weighty cream or a lot of high-fiber, crude vegetables.

Juice

Non-sweet squeeze is a great decision also. Apple and carrot juice make for a superb pick while fasting. They are high in supplements and will give you the energy you need to overcome the day without being too high in calories, making it simpler for you to get more fit when the time has come to eat once more. Notwithstanding, maintain a strategic distance from squeezed orange as it contains a great deal of sugar.

Soda

Skip it. In case you're contemplating whether you can drink soda (or diet soda) while you're doing intermittent fasting, Palinski-Wade suggests avoiding soda by and large, regardless of whether you're not after a diet like intermittent fasting. Customary sodas are generally stacked with sugar and calories and offer no dietary benefit, she says. There likewise isn't sufficient information and exploration to say whether diet soda is OK to drink during IF; however, research proposes that burning-through such a large number of fake sugars (as diet sodas will in general have) can expand desires and craving, just like advancing weight acquisition and fat capacity.

Liquor

Say no thanks to it. Liquor should never be burned-through when in a fasting period, as its belongings can be increased when burned-through on an unfilled stomach, says Palinski-Wade. Liquor is likewise a wellspring of calories, so drinking it would break your fast while additionally likely animating your craving and prompting expanded appetite and longings.

CHAPTER 17:

Various Intermittent Fasting Protocols

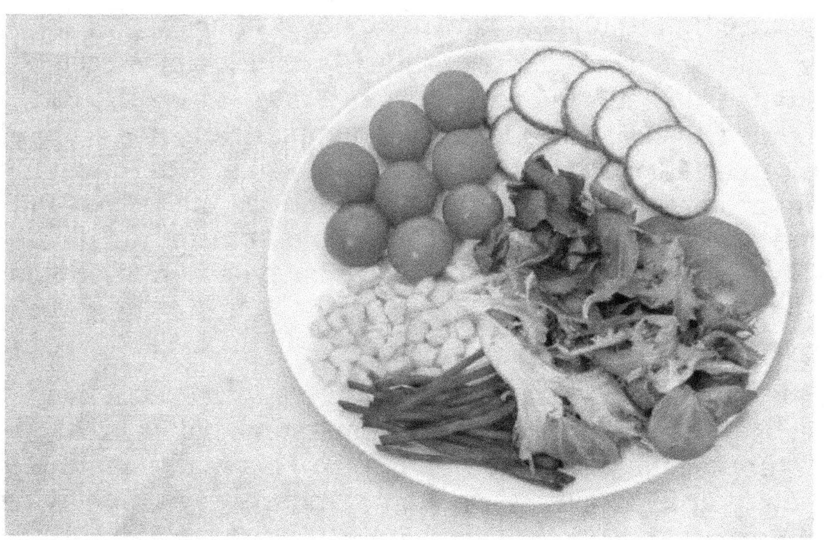

24-hour Fasting Protocol

Quite possibly the most famous intermittent fasting method–you fast for around 24 hours and have one feast soon after. Notwithstanding what the name may recommend, you will not really experience a whole day without eating. Basically, eat around night, fast all through the following day, and afterward eat again at night. The thought here is to create a caloric lack during the majority of the day, yet give one full and scrumptious supper. This method benefits most the individuals who loath eating and would prefer to have an enormous feast with all the decorations! As you progress through this method, you may conclude that a 16/8 or other method is more pleasant to your body. Individuals that do depleting exercises, for instance, will generally require additional eating windows during the day.

On the other hand, an overweight person who is mostly inactive and needs to lose some more weight could follow an intermittent fasting plan that has a larger fasting window.

36-hour Fasting Protocol

A 36-hour fast implies that you fast one whole day. You finish supper on day 1 at 7 pm, for example, and you would avoid all dinners on day 2 and not eat again until breakfast at 7 am on day 3. So that is an aggregate of 36 hours of fasting.

We will regularly suggest 36-hour fasts 2-3 times each week for type 2 diabetes in our center. As a matter of fact, this more extended fasting period creates snappier outcomes and still has great consistency. Since type 2 diabetics have more insulin obstruction, the more extended fasting time frame is more successful than more continuous more limited fasting periods, in spite of the fact that we have had great outcomes with that as well.

42-hour Fasting Protocol

We frequently encourage our customers to make an everyday practice out of skirting the morning supper and break their fast around the early afternoon hour. This makes it simple to follow a 16:8 fasting period on standard days. Following a couple of days, a great many people begin to feel very ordinary simply beginning their day with a glass of water and their typical mug of espresso.

At the point when you consolidate that with a 36-hour fast, you get a 42-hour fasting period. For instance, you would eat supper at 6 pm on day 1. You skirt all suppers on day 2 and eat your customary 'breakfast' feast at 12:00. This is a sum of 42 hours.

For longer-term fasts, we regularly make an effort NOT to limit calories during that eating period. Regularly, as individuals become accustomed to fasting, we hear all the time that their craving starts to truly go down. Not up. Down. They ought to eat to satiation on their eating day.

There's an excellent purpose behind this diminishing in craving. As you begin to break the insulin obstruction cycle, insulin levels begin to diminish. Accordingly, hunger is smothered and complete energy consumption is kept up. So, hunger goes down and TEE (Total Energy Expenditure) stays the same or goes up. Remember that ongoing ordinary caloric limitation methodologies produce the inverse. Craving goes up and TEE goes down, likely prompting substandard outcomes.

You can expand fasts any longer. The world record was 382 days (not suggested!), yet there are numerous individuals who can fast 7-14 days without trouble. In reality, the Master Cleanse utilized by Beyonce is essentially a variety of the 7-day fast, which permits some mixture of maple syrup, cayenne pepper and lemonade.

There are some hypothetical advantages of animating autophagy, a cell cleaning measure that frequently requires 48 hours of fasting or more. A condition of ketosis may need over 36 hours of fasting to enter. There are numerous hypothetical advantages, including craving concealment and greater mental clarity. For disease anticipation, some suggest a 7-day fast. In any case, a significant number of these advantages are hypothetical and troublesome. By the by, many have discovered the 7-day fast significantly less troublesome than one at first envisions.

CHAPTER 18:

Overcoming Down Moments in Fasting

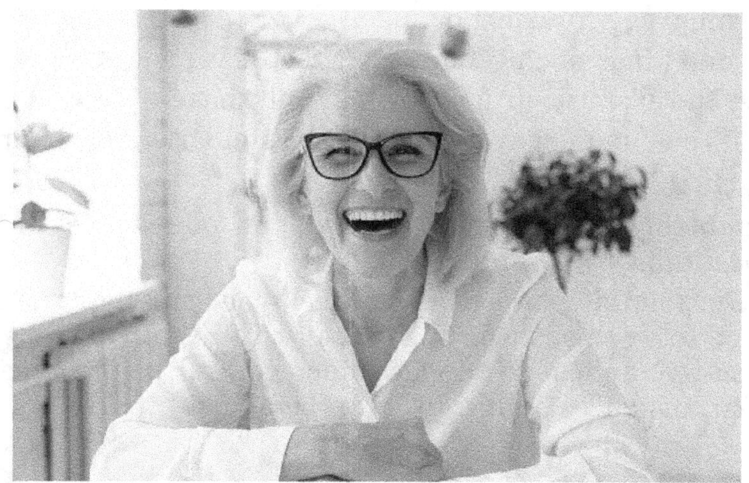

Regarding one's definitive well-being and wants to accomplish the objectives, controlling hunger and keeping sound food is significant. Intermittent fasting will assist you with achieving this, yet albeit certain people can fast with almost no issue for extended lengths, a few people can think that it's a touch really testing, especially when they first beginning.

There is a bunch of thoughts to assist you with the trip that one can use to get the best outcomes and make the ride a little smoother.

Start the Fast After Dinner

A standout amongst other guidance that can be offered is the point at which you do standard, or week after week fasting is to start the fast after supper. This strategy guarantees you will be resting for a decent bit of the fasting time, particularly when utilizing a day by day fasting method like 16:8

Eat More Satisfying Meals

The sort of food you are accustomed to influences your eagerness to both the desire to finish the fast and what you would love to eat after. An excess of pungent and sweet nourishments will make you hungrier. Instead, consume food that is enjoyable, fulfilling, and that can assist you with getting thinner, like:

• Morning: eggs or oats porridge.

• A sound lunch of chicken breast, heated yam, and veggies.

• After the exercise, drink a protein milkshake.

• Then you end the day at night with a similarly great supper.

Control Your Appetite

Undoubtedly, while fasting, cravings for food can set in from the beginning to the end.

The trick as this happens is to check your craving. The ideal method to do this is using zero-calorie refreshments that help give satiety and hold hunger under control before breaking the fast. Instances of food to control cravings are:

• Sparkling water

• Water

• Black tea

• Black espresso

• Green tea

• Herbal teas and other zero-calorie unsweetened beverages
8.4 Stay Busy

Weariness is the fundamental threat. It is the undetectable professional killer who, little by little, sneaks in to demolish the advancement, separating you consistently and hauling you downwards. Briefly, consider everything. How regularly fatigue has made you devour beyond what you can, mean to, or even realize that you are. Henceforth attempt to design your day.

Adhere to a Routine

Start and break your fast every day on customary occasions. Burning-through a diet week by week where you finish comparable things each day. Prepare supper ahead of time.

Making a routine permits to cling to the IF plan. Take out the vulnerability and re-think the interaction until you realize what works for you and focus on it consistently. Finishing it is what you need to do.

Give Yourself Time to Adjust

When one first begins intermittent fasting, chances are we will fail a few times; this is both OK and normal. It's only ordinary to have food cravings. This doesn't imply that you need to surrender or that it won't be successful for you. On the other hand, it's an opportunity to learn, to find out if or how you wrecked, and make a move to stop it from happening once more.

Live It Up

Allow yourself to appreciate the interaction. Nobody begins at the professional level, so you should go out with your companions and go to those birthday celebrations as well.

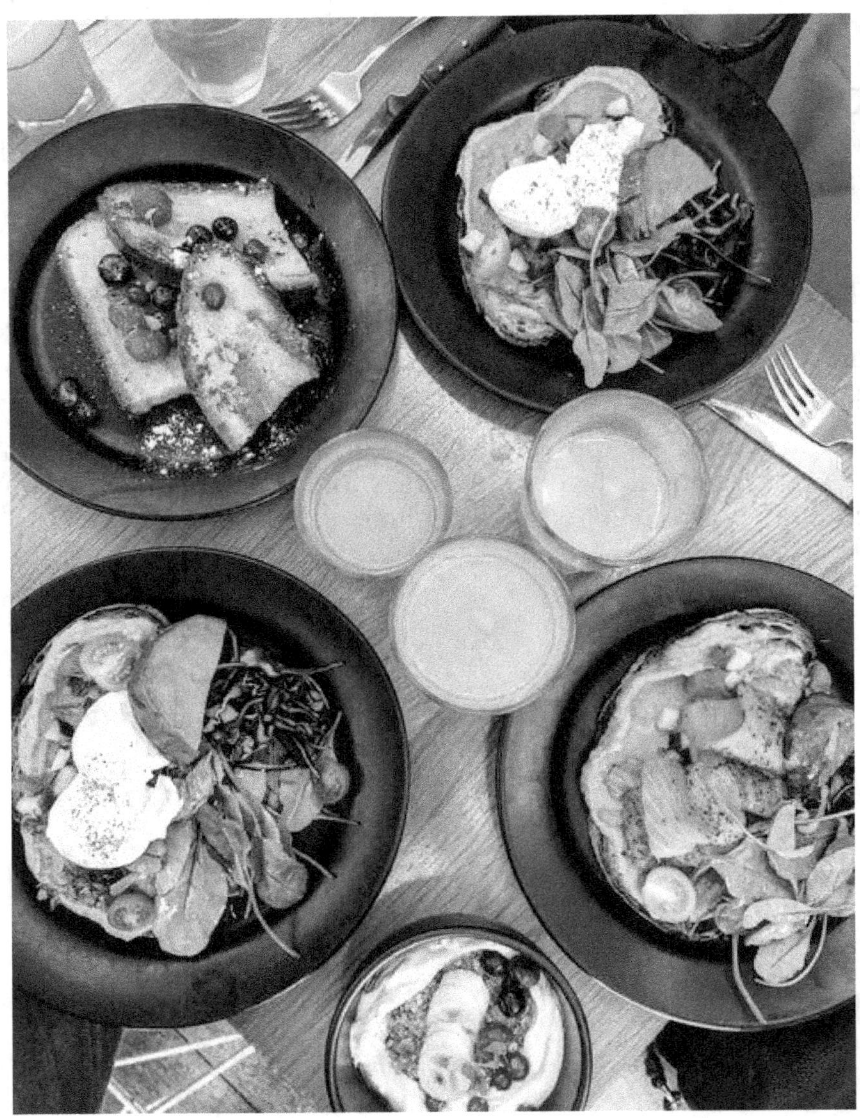

CHAPTER 19:

Recipe Book

1. Semifreddo With Berries

Preparation time: 6 h. 40 min.

Cooking time: 40 min.

Servings: 4

Ingredients:

- 2 ½ cups ripe blackberries
- 2 cups raspberries
- 1 cup sugar
- ¼ cup water
- 1 pinch salt
- 3 large egg whites
- 1 cup cream (48% cup)

Directions:

1. Line a 23cm x13cm| 9 x-5" portion tin with a twofold layer of stick film.

2. Put the blackberries and raspberries in a food processor and mix.

3. Warmth the sugar, water and salt to a bubble in a skillet, mixing until the sugar is broken down. Bubble for 2 minutes.

4. Whisk the egg whites in an enormous bowl until frothy. Gradually empty the hot sugar syrup into the egg whites, racing for 8-10 minutes, until the egg whites are cooled to room temperature.

5. Whisk the cream until thick.

6. Overlap the berry puree into the egg white combination until practically mixed, at that point overlay in the whipped cream.

7. Cover with foil and freeze for at any rate 6 hours or overnight.

8. Around 15 minutes prior to serving, eliminate the semifreddo from the cooler. Serve.

Nutrition:

- Calories: 241 Protein 3.16 g
- Fat 11.24 g Carbohydrates 34.14g
- Sugar 25.15g

2. Bulletproof Coffee

Preparation time: 5 minutes

Cooking time: 0 minutes

Servings: 1

Ingredients:

- 1 cup of brewed bulletproof coffee beans
- 1 tsp. to 2 tbsp. MCT oil
- 1-2 tbsp. grass-fed, unsalted butter

Directions:

1. Brew 1 cup (8-12 ounces) of coffee using Bulletproof coffee beans.
2. Add coffee, MCT oil and butter to a blender.
3. Blend 20-30 seconds until it looks like a creamy latte. Enjoy!

Nutrition:

- Calories: 230
- Fat: 25g
- Saturated Fat: 21g
- Carbs: 0g
- Protein: 0g
- Fiber: 0g
- Sugar: 0g
- Salt: 0mg

3. Bone Broth

Preparation time: 5 minutes
Cooking time: 4 hours
Servings: 6-8
Ingredients:
- Fish head and carcass
- 4 slices ginger
- 1 tbsp. lemon juice
- ½ leek, sliced
- Water
- Sea salt

Directions:
1. Place the fish head and carcass into a large pot with cold water.
2. Bring to a boil and pour out the water.
3. Refill the pot with fresh water and add in the leek, sea salt, ginger, and lemon juice.
4. Simmer, covered, about 4 hours.

Nutrition:
- Carbohydrates: 0 g
- Fat: 2 g
- Protein: 5 g
- Calories: 40

4. Pancakes Without Cereals

Preparation time: 10 minutes
Cooking time: 10 minutes
Servings: 2
Ingredients

- 3 ounces cream cheese
- 1 tsp ground cinnamon
- 1 tbsp honey
- 1 tsp ground cardamom
- 1 tsp butter
- 2 egg, beaten

Directions:

1. In a bowl, whisk the eggs finely.

2. Beat the cream cheese in a different bowl until it becomes soft.

3. Add the egg mixture to the softened cream cheese and mix well until there are no lumps left.

4. Add cinnamon, cardamom, and honey to it. Mix well. The batter would be runnier than of pancake batter.

5. In a pan, add the butter and heat over medium heat.

6. Add the batter using a scooper, so that all the crepe sizes would be the same.

7. Fry them golden brown on both sides.

8. Repeat the process with the rest of the batter.

9. Drizzle some honey on top and enjoy.

Nutrition:

- Calories 241
- Fats 21.8 g
- Carbohydrates 2.4g
- Proteins 9.6 g

5. Mini Omelets

Preparation time: 5 minutes
Cooking time: 15 minutes
Servings: 2
Ingredients:

- 2 cups fresh spinach leaves, already chopped
- 2 green onions, white and green parts, already sliced
- 4 large eggs
- ½ teaspoon dried oregano
- 2 tablespoons extra-virgin olive oil
- ½ cup feta cheese, crumbled and divided
- ½ cup grape tomatoes, halved
- ½ cup sliced black or Kalamata olives

Directions:

1. Warmth a huge nonstick skillet over medium-low warmth and throw in the spinach leaves and the white pieces of the green onion.

2. Add a couple of teaspoons of water and cook, blending most of the time, for 8 to 10 minutes, or until the spinach leaves are shriveled.

3. Move the spinach combination to a bowl and put it in a safe spot.

4. Eliminate the skillet from the warmth and wipe with a paper towel.

5. While the spinach is cooking, break the eggs into a bowl and add the green pieces of the green onions and the oregano. Beat softly with a fork.

6. Return the skillet to the oven, add the olive oil, and turn up the warmth to medium.

7. At the point when the oil is hot, pour in the eggs and mix delicately with the rear of a fork for 30 seconds.

8. Cook for 2 to 3 minutes or until the eggs are practically set, extricating the edges infrequently with a spatula and tenderly shifting the skillet to allow the uncooked eggs to arrive at the outside of the skillet.

9. Add the spinach blend, ¼ cup of the feta cheddar, grape tomatoes, and olives to the center of the omelet. Allow the eggs to cook for another 20 to 30 seconds until they're set.

10. Tap the handle of the dish strongly with your clenched hand to slacken the omelet and afterward overlay it over the spinach, cheddar, tomatoes, and olives with a fork or spatula.

11. Slide the omelet onto a plate and disperse the excess ¼ cup of feta cheddar up and over. Cut the omelet into equal parts and serve right away.

Replacement Tip: One (16-ounce) bundle of frozen hacked spinach can be utilized rather than new. Thaw out first by running the frozen spinach under warm water in a sifter or microwaving for 1 to 2 minutes until the spinach is delicate.

Wrap a paper towel around the spinach and press the abundance of water out over a sink.

Nutrition:

- Calories: 422
- Total fat: 36g
- Total carbs: 9g
- Fiber: 3g
- Sugar: 4g
- Protein: 20g
- Sodium: 880mg

6. Homemade Bacon

Preparation time: 2 hours

Cooking time: 5 minutes

Servings: 5

Ingredients:

- 1 lb to 2 of new pork gut the external skin ought to be eliminated. Search for pre-cut.
- Tbsp maple syrup
- Newly ground dark pepper
- Salt or smoked salt like the smoked salt best

Directions:

1. Preheat the oven to 225 degrees F.
2. Cut the pork belly to the thickness you like. I incline toward thick-cut bacon, but in the event that you need it thinner, you might need to request that your butcher cut it for you. It takes a sharp blade and a string consistent hand to do it well. Pre-cut new pork belly is likewise frequently accessible. In the case of cutting it yourself, cut the pork belly section down the middle to make more limited and simpler cuts.
3. Line an aluminum treat sheet with material paper and lay the cuts of pork belly on the paper.
4. Brush the maple syrup on one side of the pork belly cuts and sprinkle on a squeeze or two every one of salt and pepper. You are in charge of the sums here.
5. Turn the entirety of the pork belly cuts over and rehash the brushing of maple syrup and the sprinkling of salt and pepper.
6. Heat in the preheated oven for 1/2 hours for thick-cut bacon and about an hour for slender bacon. This will completely cook the meat and mellow it impressively. Turn the bacon on more than one occasion during the cooking time.
7. At this stage, you can allow it to cool to room temperature prior to putting away it in an impermeable holder in the ice chest for some time in the future.

8. To serve the bacon, heat a cast iron skillet over medium low heat and add however much bacon you wish to serve.

9. You would prefer not to cook this bacon over high heat. The lower temperature, the better is prompted for two reasons. First, the sugar substance of the maple syrup can consume on too high a heat and second, the slower it is cooked, the more fat will deliver out and the crispier your bacon will be. Thick-cut bacon can broil for 15 minutes or more under all around controlled heat.

10. At the point when firm, channel on paper towels prior to serving.

Nutrition:

- Calories: 120
- Fat: 10.6g
- Sat Fat: 1.9g
- Cholesterol: 115mg
- Sodium: 220mg
- Carbohydrates: 10g
- Sugar: 4.7g
- Protein: 4.2g

7. Grain-Free Cauliflower Pizza

Preparation time: 20 minutes
Cooking time: 42 minutes
Servings: 2
Ingredients:

For Crust:

- 1 small head cauliflower, cut into florets
- 2 large organic eggs, beaten lightly
- ½ teaspoon dried oregano
- ½ teaspoon garlic powder
- Ground black pepper, as required

For Topping:

- ½ cup sugar-free pizza sauce
- ¾ cup mozzarella cheese, shredded
- ¼ cup black olives, pitted and sliced
- 2 tablespoons Parmesan cheese, grated

Directions:

1. Preheat your oven to 400 F (200 C). Line a baking sheet with lightly greased parchment paper. Add the cauliflower in a food processor and pulse until rice-like texture is achieved.
2. In a bowl, add the cauliflower rice, eggs, oregano, garlic powder, and black pepper and mix until well combined. Place the cauliflower mixture in the center of the prepared baking sheet and press into a 13-inch thin circle with a spatula.
3. Bake for 40 minutes or until golden-brown. Remove the baking sheet from the oven. Now, set the oven to broiler on high.
4. Place the tomato sauce on top of the pizza crust and with a spatula, spread evenly and sprinkle with olives, followed by the cheeses.
5. Broil for about 1-2 minutes or until the cheese is bubbly and browned.

6. Remove from oven and with a pizza cutter, cut the pizza into equal-sized triangles. Serve hot.

Nutrition:

- **Calories**: 119
- **Fat**: 6.6g
- **Sat Fat**: 1.8g
- **Cholesterol**: 98mg
- **Sodium**: 297mg
- **Carbohydrates**: 8.6g
- **Fiber**: 3.4g
- **Sugar**: 3.7g
- **Protein**: 8.3g

8. "Breaded" Chicken in the Pork Rind

Preparation time: 18 min

Cooking time: 40 min

Servings: 2

Ingredients:

- Boneless skinless chicken breast 12 ounce (340g)
- Salt ¼ teaspoon (2g or 0.07 oz)
- Black pepper ¼ teaspoon
- Cayenne ¼ teaspoon
- Fried pork rinds 3-½ cup, whole pieces (112g or 3.95 oz)
- Parmesan cheese 1 cup, shredded (113g or 3.99 oz)
- Onion powder ¼ teaspoon - Paprika ½ teaspoon
- Raw egg ½ large (25g or 0.88 oz)

Directions:

1. Preheat an oven to 350 degrees. Slice your chicken breast(s) into thin slices. Place a piece of plastic wrap over the chicken and pound them to a ¼" thickness.

2. Pat each piece of chicken dry with a paper towel. Sprinkle the salt, pepper, and cayenne over the chicken.

3. To make the breading, pulse together the pork rinds, parmesan, paprika, and onion powder until you have a fine breading.

4. Spread the breading on a large plate and whisk together an egg in a bowl. Have this ready to go with your seasoned chicken.

5. Dip each piece of chicken one by one in the egg, shake off the excess liquid, then press into the breading. Press the chicken's bread so that it's entirely covered before setting it on a sheet tray lined with parchment paper.

6. Bake the tray for 30 minutes, flip the chicken over, and bake for an additional 10-15 minutes until done and crispy.

Nutrition:

- **Calories:** 160 **Fat:** 19g
- **Protein:** 17g**Carbs:** 1.8g

9. Chicken Legs Wrapped in Bacon

Preparation time: 10 minutes

Cooking time: 30 minutes

Servings: 4

Ingredients:

- 1 large skinless chicken breast, cut into small bites
- 9 slices bacon, cut into thirds
- 3 tbsp. garlic powder

Directions:

1. Preheat the oven to 400°F. Line a baking tray with foil.

2. Place the garlic powder in a bowl and dip each chicken piece into the garlic powder.

3. Wrap each bacon piece around each garlic chicken bite.

4. Place each bite on the baking tray, spacing them out so that they're not touching.

5. Bake for 25-30 minutes until crispy.

Nutrition:

- **Carbohydrates**: 5.3 g
- **Fat**: 5.9 g
- **Protein**: 23.5 g
- **Calories**: 170

10. Peppers Stuffed With Chicken

Preparation time: 10 minutes
Cooking time: 12 minutes
Servings:4
Ingredients:

- 4 chicken breast halves, skinless and boneless
- Salt and black pepper to taste
- 4 teaspoons olive oil
- Small cucumber, sliced
- Teaspoons cilantro, chopped
- Greek whole wheat tortillas
- Tablespoons peanut sauce

Directions:

1. Heat a grill pan over medium high heat, season chicken with salt and pepper, rub with the oil, add to the grill, cook for 6 minutes on each side, transfer to a cutting board, leave to cool down for 5 minutes, slice and leave aside.

2. In a bowl, mix cilantro with cucumber and stir.

3. Heat a pan over medium heat, add each tortilla, heat up for 20 seconds and transfer them to a working surface.

4. Spread 1 tablespoon peanut sauce on each tortilla, divide chicken and cucumber mix on each, fold, arrange on plates and serve.

Nutrition:

- **Calories**: 321
- **Fat**: 3g
- **Fiber**: 4g
- **Carbs**: 7g
- **Protein**: 9g

11.   Spiced Chicken Wings

Preparation time: 10 minutes
Cooking time: 35 minutes
Servings: 5
Ingredients:

- 2 lbs. chicken wings
- 2 tbsp. sesame oil
- ¼ cup tamari sauce
- 1 tbsp. ginger powder
- 2 tsp white wine vinegar
- 3 cloves garlic, minced
- ¼ tsp sea salt

Directions:

1. Preheat oven to 400°F.

2. In a large container, whisk together the ginger powder, sesame oil, salt, tamari sauce, vinegar, and garlic.

3. Add the wings to the mixture and stir to coat.

4. Place the wings on a lined baking sheet and bake for 30-35 minutes until golden and crispy.

5. If you want it crispier, turn on the broiler for a few minutes. Enjoy!

Nutrition:

- **Carbohydrates**: 1 g
- **Fat**: 22 g
- **Protein**: 18 g
- **Calories**: 277

12. Homemade Chicken Nuggets

Preparation time: 5 minutes

Cooking time: 20 minutes

Servings: 6

Ingredients:

- Chicken, cooked - 2 cups
- Cream cheese - 8 oz.
- Egg - 1
- Almond flour - ¼ cup
- Garlic salt - 1 teaspoon.

Directions:

1. While the chicken is still warm, set it in an electric mixer and shred. In case you are using leftover chicken, warm it up for a short period of time.

2. Once the shredding is done, add all the remaining ingredients and mix it up.

3. Drop scoops of the mixture onto a greased baking sheet, flatten it into a nugget shape.

4. Bake it for 13 minutes at 350 degrees, till they turn golden and cooked.

5. Enjoy when hot!

Nutrition:

- **Calories:** 150
- **Fat:** 18g
- **Protein:** 15g
- **Carbs:** 1.8g

13.   Beef Fajitas

Preparation time: 10 minutes
Cooking time: 3 hours
Servings: 8
Ingredients:

- 1 ½ pound beef sirloin, cut into thin strips
- 2 tablespoons lemon juice
- 2 tablespoons olive oil
- 1 garlic clove, minced
- 1 and ½ teaspoon cumin, ground
- ½ teaspoon chili powder
- A pinch of red pepper flakes, crushed
- 1 red bell pepper, cut into thin strips
- 1 yellow onion, cut into thin strips
- 8 mini coconut flour tortillas

Directions:

1. Heat a pan with the oil over medium-high heat, add beef strips, brown them for a few minutes and transfer them to your Slow cooker.

2. Add lemon juice, garlic, cumin, chili powder, and pepper flakes to the slow cooker as well, cover, and cook on High for 2 hours.

3. Add bell pepper and onion, stir and cook on High for 1 more hour. Divide the beef mix between your mini tortillas and serve for lunch.

Nutrition:

- **Calories**: 352
- **Protein**: 28.2g
- **Carbohydrates**: 18.9g
- **Fat**: 18g
- **Fiber**: 2.6g
- **Cholesterol**: 76mg
- **Sodium**: 175mg
- **Potassium**: 407mg

14. Rocket and Ham Salad

Preparation time: 5 minutes
Cooking time: 15 minutes
Servings: 4
Ingredients:

- 6 sliced ham
- 2 shallots, chopped
- 1 teaspoon olive oil
- 1/3 cup smoked ham, chopped
- 1/3 cup sweet green pepper, chopped
- 1/4 cup brie cheese
- Sea salt & black pepper to taste
- 4 Lettuce Leaves

Directions:

1. Heat the olive oil in a pan using medium heat. Add in your shallots and green pepper, letting them cook for five minutes while stirring frequently.
2. Mix all the ingredients. Serve.

Nutrition

- **Calories:** 610
- **Fat:** 21g
- **Carbs:** 10g
- **Protein:** 41g

15.   Rocket Salad With Pears and Pine Nuts

Preparation time: 5 minutes
Cooking time: 10 minutes
Servings: 3
Ingredients:

- 4 cups rocket leaves firmly packed
- 1 pear cored just ripe thinly sliced
- 1 Spanish onion thinly sliced
- 2 tbsp pine nuts roasted
- 100 g blue cheese
- 1 tsp salt and pepper
- 3 tbsp balsamic glaze
- 2 tbsp olive oil

Directions:

1. Combine rocket leaves, sliced pear, onion, pine nuts and blue vein. Season with salt and pepper to taste.

2. Drizzle balsamic glaze and a little virgin olive oil over the salad and mix gently.

Nutrition:

- **Calories**: 233
- **Fat**: 9 g
- **Fiber**: 3.5 g
- **Carbs**: 11.4 g
- **Protein**: 5.6g

16. Kale And Strawberry Salad

Preparation time: 5 minutes
Cooking time: 0 minutes
Servings: 6
Ingredients:

- 1 avocado, peeled, pitted and mashed
- 2 tablespoons almond milk
- 1 tablespoon poppy seeds
- 4 cups Kale
- 1 tablespoon balsamic vinegar
- 1 cup strawberries, sliced
- 2 tablespoons almonds, toasted and chopped

Directions:

1. In a bowl, mix the avocado with the kale and the rest of the ingredients, toss and serve for breakfast.

Nutrition:

- **Calories**: 145
- **Fat**: 1.9g
- **Fiber**: 1.2g
- **Carbs**: 3.6g
- **Protein**: 2.3g

17. Tomato, Cucumber And Avocado Salad

Preparation time: 15 minutes
Cooking time: 0 minutes
Servings: 1
Ingredients:

- 1/4 cup light mayonnaise
- 1/2 tablespoon lemon juice
- 1/2 tablespoon fresh dill, chopped
- 1/2 tablespoon chive, chopped
- 1 Avocado, chopped
- 1/4 cup feta cheese, crumbled
- Salt and pepper to taste
- 1/2 red onion, chopped
- 1/2 cucumber, diced
- 1/2 radish, diced
- 1 tomato, diced
- Chives, chopped

Directions:

1. Combine the mayonnaise, lemon juice, fresh dill, chives, feta cheese, salt, and pepper in a bowl. Mix well. Stir in the onion, cucumber, radish, avocado and tomatoes. Coat evenly. Garnish with the chopped chives.

Nutrition:

- **Calories:** 187
- **Fat:** 16.7g
- **Carbohydrates:** 6.7g
- **Protein:** 3.3g

18.   Avocado Crisps

Preparation time: 10 minutes
Cooking time: 0 minute
Servings: 2
Ingredients:

- 1 avocado, halved and pitted
- 10 ounces canned tuna, drained
- 2 tablespoons sun-dried tomatoes, chopped
- 1 and ½ tablespoon basil pesto
- 2 tablespoons black olives, pitted and chopped
- Salt and black pepper to the taste
- 2 teaspoons pine nuts, toasted and chopped
- 1 tablespoon basil, chopped

Directions:

1. In a bowl, combine the tuna with the sun-dried tomatoes and the rest of the ingredients except the avocado and stir.
2. Stuff the avocado halves with the tuna mix and serve as an appetizer.

Nutrition:

- **Calories:** 233
- **Fat:** 9 g
- **Fiber:** 3.5 g
- **Carbs:** 11.4 g
- **Protein:** 5.6

19.   Green Beans With Mustard

Preparation time: 5 minutes
Cooking time: 10 minutes
Servings: 6-8
Ingredients

- 500g French bean, trimmed
- 25g butter
- 1 shallot, finely chopped
- 1 tbsp wholegrain mustard
- 3 tbsp crème fraiche
- Juice 1 lemon

Directions:

1. Carry an enormous container of water to the bubble, at that point, drop in the green beans and cook for 4-5 minutes until they are simply cooked yet at the same time splendid green and with a slight crunch.

2. While the beans are cooking, heat the margarine in a huge shallow dish and mellow the shallot. Add the mustard and crème fraîche, and bring to a stew to join. Add the depleted beans and lemon juice, mix until equitably covered and at that point, serve straight away.

Nutrition:

- **Calories:** 130kcal
- **Fat:** 2.1
- **Fiber:** 5
- **Carbohydrates:** 21g
- **Protein:** 5 g

20.   Baked Cauliflower Rice

Cooking time: 1 hour

Servings: 8

Ingredients:

- 1 and ½ cups blackberries
- 1 cup coconut cream
- 1 tablespoon cinnamon powder
- 2 teaspoons vanilla extract
- 1 teaspoon ginger, ground
- 1 cup cauliflower rice
- ¼ cup walnuts, chopped
- 2 cups almond milk

Directions:

1. In a baking dish, combine the cauliflower rice with the berries, the cream and the other ingredients. Toss and bake at 350 degrees F for 1 hour.

2. Divide the mix into bowls and serve for breakfast.

Nutrition:

- **Calories**: 213
- **Fat**: 4.1
- **Fiber**: 4
- **Carbs**: 41
- **Protein**: 4.5

Conclusion

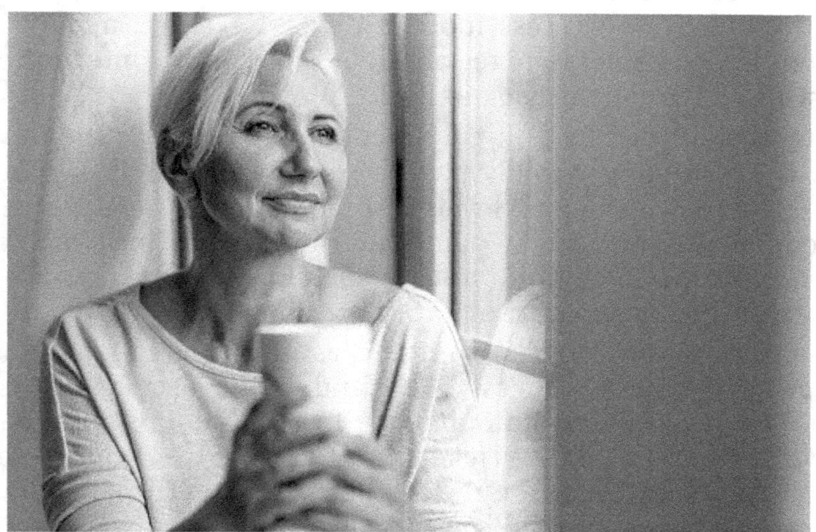

The word "intermittent" in the term intermittent fasting is hardly what comes to mind when we think of our time's dieting concept. The implication is that we are on and off diets throughout the year, without any consistency. Which is why countless individuals have given up on diets altogether.

However, what if we are wrong? What if we should actually think of intermittent fasting as a more sustainable form of diet? One that allows us to eat during specified periods throughout the day while fasting for others? This way, there could be fewer food restrictions and less hunger as you can still eat meals strategically throughout your day. One breakfast before you head to work would not mean eating nothing for most of the day until dinner.

Women over 50 have a lot to gain from intermittent fasting, as it is a time when our bodies become more susceptible to weight gain than at any other time in our lives. The most obvious reasons are that we are now entering menopause, and we may not be as active as we were when we were young. We do not need convincing that those two things put together can be disastrous in the form of excess weight, especially around the midsection. It can also "freeze" our metabolisms and make us less likely to eat less food and exercise more, making us even more vulnerable to obesity. Thankfully, intermittent fasting can break this vicious cycle.

Intermittent fasting is highly recommended for women over 50 because our thyroids may be slowing down. This means that thyroid hormone levels drop, resulting in a sluggish metabolism and weight gain. Intermittent fasting will help normalize your thyroid functions, allowing the thyroid to work optimally and improve your metabolism.

The third reason why intermittent fasting is suited for women over 50 is that it reduces cancer and cardiovascular diseases due to its cellular autophagy effects. Cellular autophagy involves cells doing housekeeping to get rid of unnecessary tissues that are clogged up with toxins. This, in turn, results in a diabetes-free metabolism. It also slows down the aging process by keeping our cells healthier for longer.

The primary takeaway is that there are numerous alternatives for ladies beyond 50 years old to assume responsibility for their weight reduction techniques without going to strategies intended for men or individuals in their twenties. Further, assuming responsibility for your wellbeing and assuming a functioning part in your illness hazard decrease isn't pretty much as troublesome as it sounds. I trust that subsequent to understanding this, you have another comprehension of what you can do and how your body will respond given your age and sex.

As you take the entirety of this data forward with you, it might appear to be overpowering to start applying this into your own life. Keep in mind, life is an interaction, and you don't have to anticipate flawlessness from yourself. By understanding this, you are already on your approach to transforming yourself.

www.ingramcontent.com/pod-product-compliance
Lightning Source LLC
Chambersburg PA
CBHW070133260726
48658CB00001B/390